T0383249

Angioedema

Editor

BRUCE L. ZURAW

IMMUNOLOGY AND ALLERGY
CLINICS OF NORTH AMERICA

www.immunology.theclinics.com

Consulting Editor
RAFEUL ALAM

November 2013 • Volume 33 • Number 4

ELSEVIER

1600 John F. Kennedy Boulevard • Suite 1800 • Philadelphia, Pennsylvania, 19103-2899

http://www.theclinics.com

IMMUNOLOGY AND ALLERGY CLINICS OF NORTH AMERICA Volume 33, Number 4

November 2013 ISSN 0889–8561, ISBN-13: 978-0-323-24225-7

Editor: Pamela Hetherington

Immunology and Allergy Clinics of North America (ISSN 0889–8561) is published quarterly by Elsevier Inc., 360 Park Avenue South, New York, NY 10010-1710. Months of issue are February, May, August, and November. Periodicals postage paid at New York, NY and additional mailing offices. Subscription prices are $320.00 per year for US individuals, $454.00 per year for US institutions, $150.00 per year for US students and residents, $395.00 per year for Canadian individuals, $220.00 per year for Canadian students, $577.00 per year for Canadian institutions, $445.00 per year for international individuals, $577.00 per year for international institutions, $220.00 per year for international students. To receive student/resident rate, orders must be accompanied by name of affiliated institution, date of term, and the *signature* of program/residency coordinator on institution letterhead. Orders will be billed at individual rate until proof of status is received. Foreign air speed delivery is included in all *Clinics* subscription prices. All prices are subject to change without notice. **POSTMASTER**: Send address changes to *Immunology and Allergy Clinics of North America*, Elsevier Health Sciences Division, Subscription Customer Service, 3251 Riverport Lane, Maryland Heights, MO 63043. **Customer Service:** 1-800-654-2452 (U.S. and Canada); 314-447-8871 (outside U.S. and Canada). Fax: 314-447-8029. E-mail: journalscustomerservice-usa@elsevier.com (for print support); journalsonlinesupport-usa@elsevier.com (for online support).

Reprints. For copies of 100 or more, of articles in this publication, please contact the Commercial Reprints Department, Elsevier Inc., 360 Park Avenue South, New York, New York 10010-1710. Tel. 212-633-3874, Fax: 212-633-3820, E-mail: reprints@elsevier.com.

Immunology and Allergy Clinics of North America is covered in MEDLINE/PubMed (Index Medicus), Current Contents/Life Sciences, Science Citation Index, ISI/BIOMED, Chemical Abstracts, and EMBASE/Excerpta Medica.

Printed and bound by CPI Group (UK) Ltd, Croydon, CR0 4YY

Transferred to digital print 2012

Contributors

CONSULTING EDITOR

RAFEUL ALAM, MD, PhD
Professor and Chief, Division of Allergy and Immunology, National Jewish Health, University of Colorado Denver School of Medicine, Denver, Colorado

EDITOR

BRUCE L. ZURAW, MD
Professor of Medicine, Division of Rheumatology, Allergy and Immunology, University of California San Diego, La Jolla, California

AUTHORS

JONATHAN A. BERNSTEIN, MD
Professor of Medicine, Allergy Section, Division of Immunology, Department of Internal Medicine, College of Medicine, University of Cincinnati, Cincinnati, Ohio

KONRAD BORK, MD
Department of Dermatology, Johannes Gutenberg University, Mainz, Germany

FLEUR BOSSI, PhD
Department of Life Sciences; Department of Medical, Surgical and Health Sciences, University of Trieste, Trieste, Italy

LAURENCE BOUILLET, MD, PhD
National Reference Centre for Angioedema (CREAK), Internal Medicine Department, Grenoble University Hospital, Joseph Fourier Grenoble 1 University, Grenoble, France

DELPHINE CHARIGNON
PhD Student, Université Joseph Fourier, GREPI/AGIM CNRS FRE 3405; French Reference Center for Angioedema, CREAK, Grenoble, France

SANDRA C. CHRISTIANSEN, MD
Clinical Professor of Medicine, Southern California Kaiser Permanente, University of California San Diego, La Jolla, California

MARCO CICARDI, MD
Department of Biological and Clinical Sciences Luigi Sacco, Ospedale Luigi Sacco, University of Milan, Milan, Italy

SVEN CICHON, PhD
Department of Genomics, Life and Brain Center, Institute of Human Genetics, University of Bonn, Germany; Division of Medical Genetics, Department of Biomedicine, University of Basel, Switzerland

FRANÇOISE CSOPAKI
Université Joseph Fourier, GREPI/AGIM CNRS FRE 3405, Grenoble, France

FEDERICA DEFENDI, PhD
Université Joseph Fourier, GREPI/AGIM CNRS FRE 3405; French Reference Center for Angioedema, CREAK, Grenoble, France

CHRISTIAN DROUET, PhD
Université Joseph Fourier, GREPI/AGIM CNRS FRE 3405; French Reference Center for Angioedema, CREAK, Grenoble, France

BERTRAND FAVIER, DVM, PhD
French Reference Center for Angioedema, CREAK, Grenoble, France

MICHAEL M. FRANK, MD
Samuel L. Katz Professor of Pediatrics, Medicine and Immunology, Duke University Medical Center, Durham, North Carolina

ARIJE GHANNAM, MD, PhD
Université Joseph Fourier, GREPI/AGIM CNRS FRE 3405; French Reference Center for Angioedema, CREAK, Grenoble, France

ANNE GOMPEL, MD, PhD
Department of Gynecology Endocrinology, Port Royal Cochin Hospital (AP-HP), Paris Descartes University, Paris, France; National Reference Centre for Angioedema (CREAK)

MOHAMMED HABIB, PhD
French Reference Center for Angioedema, CREAK, Grenoble, France

MARC A. RIEDL, MD, MS
Clinical Director - US HAEA Angioedema Center, Division of Rheumatology, Allergy and Immunology, University of California - San Diego, La Jolla, California

FRANCESCO TEDESCO, MD
Department of Life Sciences, University of Trieste, Trieste, Italy

ANDREA ZANICHELLI, MD
Department of Biological and Clinical Sciences Luigi Sacco, Ospedale Luigi Sacco, University of Milan, Milan, Italy

BRUCE L. ZURAW, MD
Professor of Medicine, San Diego VA Healthcare, University of California San Diego, La Jolla, California

Contents

AE attacks, activation of the serine proteases leads to the release of BK. Enzymes expressed on the endothelial cell membrane can metabolize BK, producing the agonist of the B1R, which can then be upregulated by proinflammatory stimuli, suggesting that the blockade of B1R and B2R, or gC1q/p33, may provide novel therapeutic targets.

Rare diseases, including hereditary angioedema, present a unique set of challenges for clinicians and investigators. The most successful way to negotiate these difficulties has been to develop collaborative efforts among physicians and with patient advocacy organizations and pharmaceutical companies. The US Hereditary Angioedema Association is a large non-profit patient advocacy organization that has been the catalyst for these types of collaborative arrangements involving hereditary angioedema. The dedication and unique structure of this patient advocacy organization has allowed it to make a substantial contribution to improving hereditary angioedema diagnosis and care.

IMMUNOLOGY AND ALLERGY CLINICS OF NORTH AMERICA

ISSUE OF RELATED INTEREST

Dermatologic Clinics July 2013 (Volume 31, Number 3)
Autoinflammatory Disorders
William Abramovits, MD, and Marcial Oquendo, MD, *Editors*

DOWNLOAD
Free App!

Review Articles
THE CLINICS

NOW AVAILABLE FOR YOUR iPhone and iPad

Foreword

Angioedema: What We Know and What We Need to Know

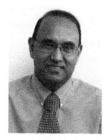

Rafeul Alam, MD, PhD
Consulting Editor

Angioedema involving airways is a life-threatening condition, which is the cause of significant morbidity, emergency room visits, and hospitalizations. The economic impact of this condition is huge. There are two major forms of angioedema—bradykinin-mediated angioedema and histamine-mediated angioedema. The bradykinin-mediated angioedema is popularly known as the complement-mediated angioedema. It is now clear that bradykinin is the final mediator of this illness regardless of the functional status of the C1 esterase inhibitor SERPING1. This conclusion is supported by genetic manipulation studies in the mouse model and the efficacy of bradykinin inhibitors in angioedema. Bradykinin-mediated angioedema can be caused by a functional deficiency of SERPING1 (type 1 and 2 hereditary angioedema), which blocks kallikrein and factor XII, the Hageman factor—the upstream activators of bradykinin. It can also be caused by mutation of the Hageman factor (type 3 hereditary angioedema). Unfortunately, many patients do not fall into either category, so they are labeled with idiopathic angioedema, although bradykinin remains the final common mediator. Bradykinin-mediated angioedema responds to treatment with the C1 esterase inhibitor (fresh frozen plasma, concentrate, or recombinant C1 esterase inhibitor), kallikrein inhibitors, and bradykinin receptor antagonists. Prophylaxis with anabolic androgens and anti-fibrinolytics is helpful. This condition contrasts with histamine-mediated angioedema, which is frequently associated with urticaria, and represents a spectrum of the urticarial syndrome. Histamine-mediated angioedema is more common than bradykinin-mediated angioedema. It can be extrinsic (allergic/IgE mediated and nonallergic), autoimmune, and idiopathic. This form of angioedema responds to antihistamines, glucocorticoids, and epinephrine.

Supported by NIH Grants RO1 AI091614 and N01 HHSN272200700048C.

http://dx.doi.org/10.1016/j.iac.2013.09.003
0889-8561/13/$ – see front matter © 2013 Published by Elsevier Inc.

immunology.theclinics.com

There are still many outstanding questions in the field of bradykinin-mediated angioedema. We need to know the mechanism of bradykinin generation in the idiopathic form of angioedema where the function of the C1 esterase inhibitor and the Hageman factor is normal. More importantly, we need a diagnostic test. We do not fully understand why C1 esterase inhibitor deficiency manifests with intermittent but not persistent angioedema. We also do not understand why patients with ACE-inhibitor-induced angioedema continue to experience symptoms weeks and months after discontinuation of the ACE-inhibitor. To update us on the pathogenesis and management of this important disease, I have invited Dr Bruce Zuraw, a leading expert in the field, to edit this very exciting issue of the *Immunology and Allergy Clinics of North America*.

Rafeul Alam, MD, PhD
Division of Allergy and Immunology
National Jewish Health and University of Colorado Denver
1400 Jackson Street
Denver, CO 80206, USA

E-mail address:
alamr@njhealth.org

Preface

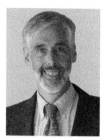

Bruce L. Zuraw, MD
Editor

It has been seven years since the last volume of *Immunology and Allergy Clinics of North America* was devoted to hereditary angioedema (HAE). Our clinical approach to and scientific understanding of HAE have significantly evolved over this time. Evaluating and treating patients with bradykinin-mediated angioedema has become substantially more complicated and requires detailed knowledge of the cause, pathophysiology, and pharmacology of the disorder. This issue attempts to summarize many of the developments in the field, reviewing what has been accomplished as well as highlighting existing areas of uncertainty.

Proper evaluation and diagnosis of patients with angioedema are essential for successful management. Most cases of angioedema are histamine-mediated; however, bradykinin-mediated or nonhistaminergic angioedema represents the most challenging cases. The differential diagnosis of recurrent nonhistaminergic angioedema has expanded and is now thought to encompass: HAE due to C1 inhibitor deficiency, type I or type II; HAE with normal C1 inhibitor, FXII or unknown types; acquired C1 inhibitor deficiency associated with anti-C1 inhibitor autoantibody and/or an underlying disease; angiotensin converting enzyme inhibitor–associated angioedema; and idiopathic nonhistaminergic angioedema. In the first article of this issue, Marco Cicardi reviews the diagnosis and evaluation of angioedema.

HAE with normal C1 inhibitor has been a disorder that has been the focus of intense investigation over the past decade. Despite even the most careful and thorough evaluation, the diagnosis of HAE with normal C1 inhibitor often remains difficult to confirm. Konrad Bork reviews the clinical picture, laboratory evaluation, genetics, and treatment of HAE with normal C1 inhibitor in our second article.

Attacks of angioedema are unpredictable and often severe and may be associated with significant morbidity or mortality. There is also substantial variability in disease severity, triggers, and response to treatment between patients. Therefore, the physician must develop a comprehensive treatment plan to manage all aspects of the disease, dealing with patient education, logistics of treatment, on-demand treatment,

Immunol Allergy Clin N Am 33 (2013) xi–xiii
http://dx.doi.org/10.1016/j.iac.2013.09.002
0889-8561/13/$ – see front matter © 2013 Published by Elsevier Inc.

and prophylaxis. In our third article, Marc Riedl reviews best practices in HAE management and outlines how to utilize evidence-based guidance documents to develop individualized HAE management plans.

Effective on-demand treatment of HAE attacks has revolutionized our approach to this disease. Over the past five years three novel therapies have been approved by the FDA for treating acute attacks of HAE and a fourth is pending approval. To be most effective, on-demand treatment must be administered early in an attack. Jonathan Bernstein reviews the on-demand treatments in our fourth article.

Long-term prophylaxis is the designation given to long-term preventive therapy to prevent attacks from occurring rather than to treat attacks that do occur. Patients who continue to experience significant disruption of their lives or morbidity despite the use of on-demand treatment may be candidates for long-term prophylaxis of HAE. The drugs available for long-term prophylaxis are very different from each other and clinicians must understand how these drugs work as well as their relative efficacy and side-effect profiles. Michael Frank in our fifth article reviews drugs available for long-term prophylaxis.

The management of HAE in women presents particular challenges because women tend to be more severely affected than men; swelling is often worsened by states of increased estrogen exposure (either endogenously and exogenously), and some of the HAE drugs are contraindicated during pregnancy and breastfeeding. Conversely, progestin therapy may be beneficial in women. Laurence Bouillet reviews the special challenges of HAE in women in our sixth article.

The major difficulty in establishing a diagnosis of HAE with normal C1 inhibitor comes from the lack of a broadly available confirmatory diagnostic test. At the current time, HAE with normal C1 inhibitor is a diagnosis of exclusion. New evidence, however, suggests that the plasma kallikrein-kinin system may be abnormal in these patients. In the seventh article, Christian Drouet reviews what is known about kallikrein-kinin system activation in HAE with normal C1 inhibitor and also suggests possible new assays that may help establish the diagnosis.

Bradykinin has been widely recognized to be the major mediator of swelling in HAE through its ability to increase vascular permeability. Most evidence has suggested that the bradykinin B2 receptor on vascular endothelial cells mediates this bradykinin-enhanced vascular permeability. More recently, some studies have suggested that the bradykinin B1 receptor may contribute significantly to bradykinin-enhanced vascular permeability. Fleur Bossi reviews this evidence in the eighth article and suggests that the bradykinin B1 receptor may be an important novel therapeutic target.

One of the biggest barriers to understanding rare diseases, including HAE, is that the rarity of the disease makes it difficult for any single investigator or even group of investigators to study large numbers of patients. In the ninth article, Bruce Zuraw describes how a proactive patient advocacy organization has partnered with HAE investigators and pharmaceutical companies to make a substantial contribution to improving HAE diagnosis and care in the United States. This type of partnership between physicians and the patient advocacy organizations can serve as a model for other rare diseases that may collectively affect up to 10% of the population.

Optimal management of HAE has undergone tremendous changes in recent years. When properly managed, most patients with HAE should now be able to live normal productive lives. Achieving this goal, however, requires that the physician understand the disease as well as the drugs that have become available to treat HAE. The articles in this issue summarize where we are in understanding and treating HAE and also suggest several areas where ongoing research may yield additional improvements in care.

Bruce L. Zuraw, MD
Division of Rheumatology, Allergy and Immunology
University of California San Diego
9500 Gilman Drive, Mailcode 0732
La Jolla, CA 92093, USA

E-mail address:
bzuraw@ucsd.edu

Diagnosing Angioedema

Marco Cicardi, MD*, Andrea Zanichelli, MD

KEYWORDS

- Angioedema • Hereditary angioedema • Diagnosis • Urticaria • Complement
- Testing

KEY POINTS

- Angioedema is a symptom, defined as a localized and self-limiting edema of the subcutaneous and submucosal tissue, caused by a temporary increase in vascular permeability. Angioedema occurs most often within the setting of allergic diseases and of different forms of urticaria. In other cases, angioedema may be a disease.
- Location of the swelling, time to development, total duration, response to therapy, and family history help distinguish, among angioedema without urticaria, histamine- and non–histamine-dependent forms and hereditary from nonhereditary angioedema.
- Nonhistaminergic forms of angioedema include hereditary angioedema.
- Evaluation of recurrent angioedema should consider specific clinical signs and appropriate laboratory findings in establishing the correct diagnosis.

Angioedema is a symptom, defined as localized and self-limiting edema of the subcutaneous and submucosal tissue, caused by a temporary increase in vascular permeability. Most often it occurs within the setting of allergic diseases and of different forms of urticaria, but situations occur in which angioedema itself represents a disease. Quinke[1] was the first author who gave a separate description of these "circumscribed edema," which he called "angioneurotic edema." Shortly after Quinke, Osler,[2] in his seminal paper "Hereditary Angioneurotic Edema," gave the first exhaustive description of an angioedema as a separate nosologic entity.

Until the end of the 20th century, hereditary angioneurotic edema, renamed *hereditary angioedema* (HAE) by Rosen and Austen,[3] remained synonymous with hereditary deficiency of C1 inhibitor, the first biochemical defect identified to cause a recurrent form of angioedema.[4] In 2000, Bork and colleagues[5] described a series of families with a new form of HAE characterized by normal C1 inhibitor. From that point on, properly diagnosing a recurrent angioedema became a significant problem for the physician.

Department of Biological and Clinical Sciences Luigi Sacco, Ospedale Luigi Sacco, University of Milan, Milano, Italy
* Corresponding author.
E-mail address: marco.cicardi@unimi.it

Immunol Allergy Clin N Am 33 (2013) 449–456
http://dx.doi.org/10.1016/j.iac.2013.07.001
0889-8561/13/$ – see front matter © 2013 Elsevier Inc. All rights reserved.
immunology.theclinics.com

In 2013, a physician who sees a patient for recurrent angioedema must consider specific clinical and laboratory signs to properly frame the patient and prepare a therapeutic plan.

CLINICAL DIAGNOSIS

The first clinical issue to be considered is presence or absence of concomitant wheals, which distinguishes urticaria from angioedema. Classification of urticaria was recently summarized, and angioedema occurring as part of the urticaria follows the same classification.[6,7] Location, time to development, total duration, and family history help to distinguish, among angioedema without urticaria, histamine- from non–histamine-dependent types and hereditary from nonhereditary angioedema (**Tables 1** and **2**). Recurrent abdominal pain due to temporary bowel occlusion caused by swelling within the gastrointestinal mucosa[8] is characteristic of HAE with and without C1 inhibitor deficiency, and of angioedema caused by acquired deficiency of C1 inhibitor. Oral and perioral location of angioedema is almost the rule in angioedema related to angiotensin-converting enzyme (ACE) inhibitors. Angioedema of the lips, or of half of them, is a frequent presentation for histaminergic forms, such as those prevented by H_1 antihistamine. These occurrences of angioedema are announced by local pruritic dysesthesia, peak rapidly within one or 2 hours, subside in 12 to 36 hours, and rarely affect the larynx.[7–9]

The relationship between angioedema and causative/facilitative factors is important to recognize. The presence of a clear chronologic cause-and-effect relationship is cardinal to diagnosing allergic angioedema, which, by definition, occur within a few hours, frequently minutes, of exposure to the offending agent. The same is true for most angioedema related to drugs, such as antibiotics or nonsteroidal anti-inflammatory drugs. More challenging is the identification of ACE inhibitors as a

Table 1
Clinical characteristics of different types of recurrent angioedema without wheals

	C1-INH HAE[a]	FXII HAE[b]	UNKN HAE[c]	Histam AE[d]	Non-Histam AE[e]	C1-INH AAE[f]	ACEi AE[g]
Peripheral angioedema	+++	+++	+++	+	+	++	+−
Tongue angioedema	+	+	+	++	++	++	+++
Laryngeal angioedema	+++	+++	+++	+	+	+++	+++
Gastrointestinal angioedema	+++	+++	+++	+−	+−	++	+−
Estrogen sensitivity	++	+++	+	−	−	−	−
Onset <6 h	+	+	+	+++	++	+	++
Duration >48 h	+++	+++	+++	+	+	+++	++
Family members with angioedema	+++	+	+++	−	−	−	−

[a] Hereditary angioedema with C1 inhibitor deficiency.
[b] Hereditary angioedema with a mutation in factor XII.
[c] Hereditary angioedema with an unknown defect.
[d] Recurrent, nonfamilial angioedema of undetermined origin (idiopathic) prevented by H_1 antihistamine treatment.
[e] Recurrent, nonfamilial angioedema of undetermined origin (idiopathic) not prevented by H_1 antihistamine treatment.
[f] Recurrent angioedema with nonfamilial (acquired) C1 inhibitor deficiency.
[g] Recurrent nonfamilial angioedema onset during treatment with angiotensin-converting enzyme inhibitors.

Table 2
Laboratory characteristics of different types of recurrent angioedema without wheals

Parameter	C1-INH HAE[a]	FXII HAE[b]	UNKN HAE[c]	Histam AE[d]	Non-Histam AE[e]	C1-INH AAE[f]	ACEi AE[g]
C1 inhibitor function <50% of normal	100%	0	0	0	0	100%	0
C1 inhibitor antigen <50% of normal	85%	0	0	0	0	85%	0
C4 antigen <12 mg/dL	>90%	Occasional	Occasional	Occasional	Occasional	>90%	Occasional
C1q antigen <50% of normal	Occasional	0	0	0	0	>70%	0
Mutation in SERPING1	>90%[h]	0	0	0	0	0	0
Mutation in FXII gene	0	100%	0	0	0	0	0

Percentage of patients carrying a specific parameter is derived from the literature reported in the text and from the authors' personal experience.
[a] Hereditary angioedema with C1 inhibitor deficiency.
[b] Hereditary angioedema with mutation in factor XII.
[c] Hereditary angioedema with unknown defect.
[d] Recurrent, nonfamilial angioedema of undetermined origin (idiopathic) prevented by H_1 antihistamine treatment.
[e] Recurrent, nonfamilial angioedema of undetermined origin (idiopathic) not prevented by H_1 antihistamine treatment.
[f] Recurrent angioedema with nonfamilial (acquired) C1 inhibitor deficiency.
[g] Recurrent nonfamilial angioedema onset during treatment with angiotensin-converting enzyme inhibitors.
[h] Genetic screening in patients with hereditary C1 inhibitor deficiency fails to identify a causative mutation in 3% to 8% of the patients, depending on the methodological approach.

cause of angioedema.[10] These drugs likely facilitate angioedema in patients who are slow bradykinin catabolizers.[11,12] In these patients, angioedema rarely occurs despite continued ACE inhibitor treatment, which frequently leads to delayed identification of the relationship between angioedema and the drug when this does occur. Therefore, a careful pharmacologic history should always be obtained for patients presenting with angioedema. The fact that a treatment was started years before onset of symptoms does not rule out a potential relationship; this is always true for ACE inhibitors, and should also be considered in patients taking estrogens, which is another treatment that may affect angioedema. In addition to relatively rare instances in which estrogens directly cause angioedema, this treatment frequently worsens angioedema with and without C1 inhibitor deficiency.[13,14] Identifying the close relationship between the occurrence of angioedema and elevated estrogen levels from pregnancy or estrogen-containing pills can be nearly diagnostic for HAE with mutations in factor XII.[15]

Accurate recording of family history may be the only tool for diagnosing HAE, because HAE is not limited to the hereditary deficiency of C1 inhibitor or the presence of mutations in factor XII, but can be inherited in the absence of an identified genetic or biochemical marker.[16] This familial HAE seems to be still transmitted as an autosomal dominant trait, the same identified by Crowder and Crowder in 1917[17] for the form subsequently related to mutations in the C1 inhibitor gene.[18,19] HAE with normal C1 inhibitor and no mutations in factor XII is estimated to represent approximately 70% of the hereditary forms that are not related to C1 inhibitor deficiency. Hence, diagnosis of HAE with normal C1 inhibitor and absence of factor XII mutations is purely dependent on clinical evidence of a family history of angioedema. Determining the presence of angioedema within the family is not always straightforward, particularly when dealing with abdominal symptoms and cutaneous manifestations ranging between angioedema and urticaria. Approximately half of the general population will experience at least a single urticarial eruption. Therefore, physicians should carefully distinguish sporadic manifestations from a true family history of recurrent angioedema. Distribution of symptoms according to an autosomal mode of inheritance reinforce the finding, but the number of family members available for evaluation may be a limiting factor preventing conclusive diagnosis.

Clinical penetrance of a genetic abnormality is another factor that may affect family history. The 2 forms of angioedema that have been related to a specific genetic defect significantly differ in this respect, with C1 inhibitor deficiency having a penetrance approaching 100%, and factor XII mutations remaining clinically silent in men, and sometimes also not expressed in female carriers.[20] In families in which inheritance has not yet been related to a specific marker, penetrance obviously cannot be evaluated.

LABORATORY DIAGNOSIS

The measurement of C1 inhibitor is the core laboratory test for angioedema diagnosis. Deficiency of C1 inhibitor is the abnormality that best accounts for the presence of recurrent angioedema. It is mandatory to screen for C1 inhibitor deficiency all patients with angioedema without wheals whose symptoms do not subside during antihistamine treatment, including those who become symptomatic during ACE inhibitor or estrogen treatment. It is not uncommon for these drugs to induce the clinical expression of an underlying C1 inhibitor deficiency that has remained silent.[21,22] However, screening for C1 inhibitor deficiency is not univocally defined. Direct identification of all deficient patients requires the determination of C1 inhibitor function, because hereditary and acquired deficiency of this protein may be characterized by the presence of protein products detected by quantitative methods but devoid of functional activity. Dysfunctional C1 inhibitor is detected in approximately 15% of both hereditary and acquired C1 inhibitor deficiency (Marco Cicardi, personal case list). Two methods are currently available to measure C1 inhibitor function, and neither is routinely performed in diagnostic laboratories.[23] Both methods are based on measurement of the capacity of plasma to inhibit the esterase activity of a fixed amount of C1 esterase, quantified by chromogenic or immunoenzymatic assay. The chromogenic assay has higher specificity than the immunoenzymatic assay, whose normal values must be established by each laboratory to properly diagnose C1 inhibitor deficiency.

Measurement of C1 inhibitor and C4 antigen, routinely performed in most laboratories, can partially overcome the problem of diagnosing C1 inhibitor deficiency when the functional assay is not available. C1 inhibitor antigen fewer than 50% of normal diagnoses 85% of the deficiencies. The value of C4 measurement is indicated by the fact that C1 inhibitor deficiency causes hyperactivation of the classical complement pathway and C4 consumption. Thus, very few patients with C1 inhibitor deficiency (<10% in the authors' case list) have C4 plasma levels greater than 12 mg/dL. The high variability of the levels of this protein in the normal population, and the several diseases that may lead to C4 consumption (eg, systemic lupus erythematosus, cryoglobulinemia), reduce the specificity of this measurement. Nevertheless, levels of C4 greater than 12 mg/dL make the diagnosis of C1 inhibitor deficiency very unlikely.

When the diagnosis of C1 inhibitor deficiency has been established, measurement of the plasma levels of C1q may help distinguish between hereditary and acquired deficiency: this subcomponent of the C1 complex is almost always normal in HAE and very low in 70% of the acquired deficiencies.[24] Changes in several proteins of the contact, coagulation, and fibrinolytic systems have been identified during angioedema symptoms in patients with C1 inhibitor deficiency.[25–28] However, none of these parameters has yet achieved diagnostic value.

Genetic testing is the sole laboratory approach for diagnosing factor XII HAE. Three mutations—2 different missense mutations of codon p.Thr328 and the deletion of 72 base pairs located in the same factor XII gene region—have been shown to segregate with family symptoms of angioedema.[29] One of these mutations (Arg328Lys) accounts for most of the factor XII-HAE families described to date.[30–32] Sequencing of the short region of factor XII containing all mutations causing HAE is therefore enough for the genetic diagnosis of this type of angioedema. The controversial evidence of the effect of these mutations on factor XII activity prevents biochemical assays from being helpful in diagnosis.[33,34]

Genetic testing is less compelling for diagnosing HAE and C1 inhibitor deficiency; diagnosis usually occurs when combining biochemical findings and family history. Genetic testing is limited to situations in which a single member of the family has angioedema symptoms and C1 inhibitor deficiency, and distinction between acquired and genetic deficiency is not clear-cut. In these circumstances, the genetic basis of the disease can only be demonstrated with the evidence that the C1 inhibitor gene (SERPING1) carries a mutation preventing circulation of a normal protein in plasma. Most C1 inhibitor HAE families have so-called private mutations (ie, each family has its own mutation), and more than 300 different mutations have been associated to genetic C1 inhibitor deficiency.[35–38] Genetic diagnosis of C1 inhibitor deficiency is therefore complicated and is achieved through sequencing a preidentified mutated region in SERPING1 or all exons and exon/intron boundaries.

No biochemical or genetic marker can identify other types of angioedema. Tryptase, as marker of mast cell degranulation, could help identifying histamine-mediated angioedema, but it is not used in clinical practice because of the high number of false-negative results. Very limited help comes from allergy testing, which confirms diagnosis only when a causative agent was previously identified.

In conclusion, distinguishing between angioedema and urticaria is important for determining an appropriate therapeutic approach. Careful evaluation of the clinical clues, along with proper C1 inhibitor and genetic testing, provide the major insights for correct diagnosis.

REFERENCES

1. Quinke H. Uber akutes umschriebened hautodem. Monatshe Prakt Dermatol 1882;1:129–31.
2. Osler W. Hereditary angio-neurotic oedema. Am J Med Sci 1888;95:362–7.
3. Rosen FS, Austen KF. The "neurotic edema" (hereditary angioedema). N Engl J Med 1969;280:1356–7.
4. Donaldson VH, Evans RR. A biochemical abnormality in hereditary angioneurotic edema: absence of serum inhibitor of C' 1-esterase. Am J Sci 1963;31:37–44.
5. Bork K, Barnstedt SE, Koch P, et al. Hereditary angioedema with normal C1-inhibitor activity in women. Lancet 2000;356:213–7.
6. Zuberbier TA. Summary of the new international EAACI/GA2LEN/EDF/WAO guidelines in urticaria. World Allergy Organ J 2012;5(Suppl 1):S1–5.
7. Sanchez-Borges M, Asero R, Ansotegui IJ, et al. Diagnosis and treatment of urticaria and angioedema: a worldwide perspective. World Allergy Organ J 2012; 5:125–47.
8. Zingale LC, Zanichelli A, Deliliers DL, et al. Successful resolution of bowel obstruction in a patient with hereditary angioedema. Eur J Gastroenterol Hepatol 2008;20:583–7.
9. Kaplan AP, Greaves MW. Angioedema. J Am Acad Dermatol 2005;53:373–88 [quiz: 89–92].
10. Beltrami L, Zingale LC, Carugo S, et al. Angiotensin-converting enzyme inhibitor-related angioedema: how to deal with it. Expert Opin Drug Saf 2006;5:643–9.
11. Duan QL, Nikpoor B, Dube MP, et al. A variant in XPNPEP2 is associated with angioedema induced by angiotensin I-converting enzyme inhibitors. Am J Hum Genet 2005;77:617–26.
12. La Corte AL, Carter AM, Rice GI, et al. A functional XPNPEP2 promoter haplotype leads to reduced plasma aminopeptidase P and increased risk of ACE inhibitor-induced angioedema. Hum Mutat 2011;32:1326–31.
13. Caballero T, Farkas H, Bouillet L, et al. International consensus and practical guidelines on the gynecologic and obstetric management of female patients with hereditary angioedema caused by C1 inhibitor deficiency. J Allergy Clin Immunol 2012;129:308–20.
14. Binkley KE, Davis A 3rd. Clinical, biochemical, and genetic characterization of a novel estrogen-dependent inherited form of angioedema. J Allergy Clin Immunol 2000;106:546–50.
15. Bork K. Diagnosis and treatment of hereditary angioedema with normal C1 inhibitor. Allergy Asthma Clin Immunol 2010;6:15.
16. Zuraw BL, Bork K, Binkley KE, et al. Hereditary angioedema with normal C1 inhibitor function: consensus of an international expert panel. Allergy Asthma Proc 2012;33(Suppl 1):S145–56.

17. Crowder JR, Crowder TR. Five generations of angioneurotic edema. Arch Intern Med 1917;20:840–52.
18. Cicardi M, Igarashi T, Kim MS, et al. Restriction fragment length polymorphism of the C1 inhibitor gene in hereditary angioneurotic edema. J Clin Invest 1987;80: 1640–3.
19. Stoppa-Lyonnet D, Tosi M, Laurent J, et al. Altered C1 inhibitor genes in type I hereditary angioedema. N Engl J Med 1987;317:1–6.
20. Bork K. Hereditary angioedema with normal c1 inhibition. Curr Allergy Asthma Rep 2009;9:280–5.
21. Ricketti AJ, Cleri DJ, Ramos-Bonner LS, et al. Hereditary angioedema presenting in late middle age after angiotensin-converting enzyme inhibitor treatment. Ann Allergy Asthma Immunol 2007;98:397–401.
22. Cicardi M, Johnston DT. Hereditary and acquired complement component 1 esterase inhibitor deficiency: a review for the hematologist. Acta Haematol 2012;127:208–20.
23. Wagenaar-Bos IG, Drouet C, Aygoren-Pursun E, et al. Functional C1-inhibitor diagnostics in hereditary angioedema: assay evaluation and recommendations. J Immunol Methods 2008;338:14–20.
24. Zingale LC, Castelli R, Zanichelli A, et al. Acquired deficiency of the inhibitor of the first complement component: presentation, diagnosis, course, and conventional management. Immunol Allergy Clin North Am 2006;26:669–90.
25. Cugno M, Cicardi M, Bottasso B, et al. Activation of the coagulation cascade in C1-inhibitor deficiencies. Blood 1997;89:3213–8.
26. Cugno M, Zanichelli A, Bellatorre AG, et al. Plasma biomarkers of acute attacks in patients with angioedema due to C1-inhibitor deficiency. Allergy 2009;64:254–7.
27. Cugno M, Zanichelli A, Foieni F, et al. C1-inhibitor deficiency and angioedema: molecular mechanisms and clinical progress. Trends Mol Med 2009;15:69–78.
28. van Geffen M, Cugno M, Lap P, et al. Alterations of coagulation and fibrinolysis in patients with angioedema due to C1-inhibitor deficiency. Clin Exp Immunol 2012; 167:472–8.
29. Bork K, Wulff K, Meinke P, et al. A novel mutation in the coagulation factor 12 gene in subjects with hereditary angioedema and normal C1-inhibitor. Clin Immunol 2011;141:31–5.
30. Bork K. Hereditary angioedema with normal C1 inhibitor activity including hereditary angioedema with coagulation factor XII gene mutations. Immunol Allergy Clin North Am 2006;26:709–24.
31. Marcos C, Lopez Lera A, Varela S, et al. Clinical, biochemical, and genetic characterization of type III hereditary angioedema in 13 Northwest Spanish families. Ann Allergy Asthma Immunol 2012;109:195–200.e2.
32. Vitrat-Hincky V, Gompel A, Dumestre-Perard C, et al. Type III hereditary angiooedema: clinical and biological features in a French cohort. Allergy 2010;65: 1331–6.
33. Cichon S, Martin L, Hennies HC, et al. Increased activity of coagulation factor XII (Hageman factor) causes hereditary angioedema type III. Am J Hum Genet 2006; 79:1098–104.
34. Bork K, Kleist R, Hardt J, et al. Kallikrein-kinin system and fibrinolysis in hereditary angioedema due to factor XII gene mutation Thr309Lys. Blood Coagul Fibrinolysis 2009;20(5):325–32.
35. Rijavec M, Korosec P, Silar M, et al. Hereditary angioedema nationwide study in Slovenia reveals four novel mutations in SERPING1 gene. PLoS One 2013;8: e56712.

36. Firinu D, Colomba P, Manconi PE, et al. Identification of a novel and recurrent mutation in the SERPING1 gene in patients with hereditary angioedema. Clin Immunol 2013;147:129–32.
37. Bygum A, Fagerberg CR, Ponard D, et al. Mutational spectrum and phenotypes in Danish families with hereditary angioedema because of C1 inhibitor deficiency. Allergy 2011;66:76–84.
38. Gosswein T, Kocot A, Emmert G, et al. Mutational spectrum of the C1INH (SERPING1) gene in patients with hereditary angioedema. Cytogenet Genome Res 2008;121:181–8.

Hereditary Angioedema with Normal C1 Inhibitor

Konrad Bork, MD

KEYWORDS

- Hereditary angioedema with normal C1 inhibitor • Hereditary angioedema type III
- Coagulation factor XII • Kallikrein-kinin pathway • Mutations in the *F12* gene

KEY POINTS

- A hereditary angioedema with normal C1 inhibitor (HAE type III) should be considered if 2 or more patients per family with recurrent angioedema and normal C1 inhibitor are identified.
- The disease affects mostly women, mainly in high estrogen states, like intake of oral contraceptives and pregnancy.
- Two subgroups of hereditary angioedema with normal C1 inhibitor can be differentiated, one with a mutation in the gene encoding coagulation factor XII (HAE-FXII) and one without such a mutation (HAE-unknown).
- Hereditary angioedema with normal C1 inhibitor has an autosomal-dominant inheritance.

INTRODUCTION

Hereditary angioedema (HAE) is characterized by recurrent edema episodes in various organs, leading predominantly to skin swellings, abdominal pain attacks, and potentially life-threatening laryngeal edema. Until recently, it was assumed that HAE constitutes a single disease entity and that all patients have a genetically determined deficiency of C1-esterase inhibitor (C1-INH) due to mutations in the gene coding for C1-INH. In acute attacks in patients with HAE due to C1-INH deficiency (HAE-C1-INH), the kallikrein-kinin system (KKS) is activated, with production of bradykinin at the end of the cascade. The coagulation factor FXII (Hageman factor) is assumed to play a central role in early activation steps of the KKS.

In 2000, a novel type of HAE was described that was not associated with C1-INH deficiency and occurred mainly in women.[1] Ten families with this disease were reported. In these families a total of 36 women, but not one man, were affected with recurrent angioedema. All patients had normal C1-INH concentration and activity with respect to C1 esterase inhibition, ruling out both types of HAE (HAE type I and

Department of Dermatology, Johannes Gutenberg University, Langenbeckstr. 1, 55131 Mainz, Germany
E-mail address: bork@hautklinik.klinik.uni-mainz.de

Immunol Allergy Clin N Am 33 (2013) 457–470
http://dx.doi.org/10.1016/j.iac.2013.07.002
0889-8561/13/$ – see front matter © 2013 Elsevier Inc. All rights reserved.

immunology.theclinics.com

HAE type II).[1] In the same year, an additional family was described, with 7 affected women.[2,3] This hitherto unknown disease was proposed to be termed as *"hereditary angioedema with normal C1 inhibitor"* (HAEnCI) or "hereditary angioedema type III".[1] In a recent consensus of an international expert panel it was recommended to use the name "hereditary angioedema with normal C1-INH".[4] HAEnCI is autosomally inherited with incomplete phenotypical penetrance.[1]

In 2006, 2 different missense mutations in a nonconservative gene region were identified in German patients, located in exon 9 of the gene coding for the coagulation factor XII (Hageman factor).[5] The point mutations c.1032C>A (p.Thr328Lys) (old nomenclature: p.Thr309Lys) were observed in 5 unrelated families and the mutations c.1032C>G (p.Thr328Arg) (old nomenclature: p.Thr309Arg) were observed in one family. In 2011 a further HAE mutation was identified, a large deletion of 72 base pairs (c.971_1018+24del72).[6]

Until now, numerous families have been reported that include members having HAE with normal C1-INH, with affected women bearing these mutations (**Table 1**).

In most families with HAEnCI patients, a mutation in the *F12* gene could not be found. The author have proposed the name "HAE-unknown" for this variant of disease.[7] Therefore 2 subgroups of HAEnCI can be differentiated, HAEnCI with one of the 3 known mutations in the coagulation factor XII gene (HAE-FXII) and HAEnCI without a mutation in the *F12* gene (HAE-unknown) (**Box 1**).

CLINICAL PRESENTATION
Clinical Symptoms

The clinical symptoms of HAEnCI include recurrent skin swellings, abdominal pain attacks, tongue swellings, and laryngeal edema. In 2000, it was reported that 36 patients had relapsing skin swellings and/or attacks of abdominal pain and/or recurrent laryngeal edema.[1] Urticaria did not occur at any time in any of these patients. The skin swellings lasted 2 to 5 days; they affected mainly the extremities and the face and affected and the trunk less frequently. The abdominal attacks likewise lasted 2 to 5 days and were manifested as severe cramplike pains. In a more recent study, a total of 138 patients with HAEnCI who belonged to 43 unrelated families were examined.[8] Most patients had skin swellings (92.8%), tongue swellings (53.6%), and abdominal pain attacks (50%). Laryngeal edema (25.4%) and uvular edema (21.7%) also were frequent, whereas edema episodes of other organs were rare (3.6%). Facial swellings and tongue involvement occurred considerably more frequently compared with HAE-C1-INH. The number of patients with recurrent edema of only one organ was higher than in HAE-C1-INH. Erythema marginatum was not observed. Hence, HAEnCI shows a characteristic pattern of clinical symptoms. There are many differences in the clinical symptoms and course of disease between HAEnCI and HAE-C1-INH (**Box 2**).

The clinical manifestation of HAEnCI is highly variable, and penetrance of the disease might be low; thus, obligate female carriers, even in their seventh decade, without any clinical symptoms were observed.[1,9] Therefore, a considerable number of asymptomatic carriers may exist in the population.

Death by asphyxiation due to upper airway obstruction

In a patient series described in 2007,[8] one woman asphyxiated at the age of 16 during her first laryngeal edema attack. A second woman asphyxiated at the age of 36 after 10 episodes of upper airway obstruction, a third at the age of 38 during her eighth airway attack, and a fourth at the age of 48 after a tongue swelling.

Table 1
Hereditary angioedema with mutations in the coagulation factor XII gene: Number of families reported until now, mutations, and gender of patients

	Reported Families with HAE-FXII	Families with the p.Thr328Lys Mutation in the Factor XII Gene	Families with the p.Thr328Arg Mutation in the Factor XII Gene	Families with the Deletion Mutation in the Factor XII Gene	Number of Women Clinically Affected with HAE-FXII	Number of Men Clinically Affected with HAE-FXII
Dewald & Bork,[5] 2006	6	5	1	0	23	0
Cichon et al,[18] 2006	1	1	0	0	4	0
Bouillet et al,[19] 2007	1	1	0	0	2	0
Martin et al,[16] 2007	1	1	0	0	2	2
Bell et al,[20] 2008	1	1	0	0	1	0
Prieto et al,[21] 2009	1	1	0	0	4	0
Duan et al,[22] 2009	1	1	0	0	7	0
Nagy et al,[23] 2009	1	1	0	0	3	0
Hentges et al,[24] 2009	1	1	0	0	2	0
Bork et al,[7] 2009, further families	7	6	1	0	30	0
Picone et al,[25] 2010	2	2	0	0	3	0
Vitrat-Hincky et al,[26] 2010	3	3	0	0	6 (?)	0 (?)
Baeza et al,[27] 2011	1	1	0	0	3	0
Bork et al,[6] 2011	1	0	0	1	2	0
Marcos et al,[17] 2012	13	13	0	0	26	3

Box 1
Classification of hereditary angioedema

I. Hereditary angioedema due to C1 inhibitor deficiency (HAE-C1-INH)

    A. Type I (low C1 inhibitor activity and concentration in plasma)

    B. Type II (low C1 inhibitor activity but normal or increased C1 inhibitor concentration in plasma)

II. Hereditary angioedema with normal C1 inhibitor (HAEnCl, HAE type III)

    A. Hereditary angioedema with one of the known mutations in exon 9/intron 9 of the coagulation factor XII gene (Thr328Lys or Thr328Arg or the large deletion) (HAE-FXII)

    B. Hereditary angioedema without one of the known mutations in exon 9/intron 9 of the coagulation factor XII gene (HAE-unknown)

Onset of clinical symptoms

In a series of 138 patients, the mean age at onset of the disease was 26.8 years (SD ± 14.9 years, range 1–68 years).[8] Onset of clinical symptoms occurred in the first decade of life in 11 (8%) patients, in the second decade in 60 (43.5%) patients, in the third decade in 22 (15.9%) patients, and later in 45 (32.6%) patients. Hence, the number of patients with disease onset in adulthood was significantly higher in HAEnCl compared with HAE-C1-INH.

Box 2
Features of hereditary angioedema with normal C1-INH that serves to differentiate it from hereditary angioedema due to C1-INH deficiency

- Patients have normal C1-INH protein and activity.
- Mainly women are clinically affected.
- The number of children already affected before the age of 10 years is low. Clinical symptoms start in adulthood in more patients than in hereditary angioedema because of C1-INH deficiency.
- There are more disease-free intervals during the course of the disease.
- Symptoms are less frequent compared with hereditary angioedema because of C1-INH deficiency.
- Facial swellings, mainly lip swellings, are relatively more frequent.
- The tongue is considerably more often affected: Recurrent tongue swelling is more common than in HAE because of C1-INH deficiency.
- Many patients have only skin swellings.
- Many patients have only recurrent skin swellings and tongue swellings.
- Abdominal attacks are less frequent.
- Suffocation may be preceded and caused by a tongue swelling.
- There is no erythema marginatum (gyrated erythematous rash) as is highly characteristic of HAE because of C1-INH deficiency.
- Hemorrhages into skin swellings were observed in hereditary angioedema with normal C1-INH.

POTENTIALLY PROVOKING FACTORS
Role of Estrogens

In many women clinical symptoms either begin or are exacerbated after the intake of oral contraceptives (OC) or hormone replacement therapy (HRT) or during pregnancy.[1–3,9] Binkley and Davis[2,10] observed patients with typical symptoms of recurrent angioedema that were restricted to conditions of high estrogen levels (estrogen-dependent HAE). However, in an analysis of 228 angioedema patients receiving OC or HRT, it was demonstrated that in only 24 (62%) of 39 women with HAEnCI were the clinical symptoms induced or exacerbated after starting OCs or HRT; correspondingly, 15 (38%) of 39 women tolerated exogenous estrogens without any influence on their disease.[9] It was shown that estrogens play a considerable role in most women with HAE-FXII.[7] However, the influence of estrogens is variable (**Table 2**). The negative influence of estrogens is also well known in HAE-C1-INH and, therefore, not a specific sign for HAEnCI.

The reason for the negative impact of estrogens in HAE-FXII remains unclear. Binkley and Davis[2] also sequenced the 5′ regulatory region of factor XII gene because it contains a known estrogen response element. However, they found no abnormalities in that region in families with the p.Thr328Arg mutation in the factor XII gene.

Angiotensin-Converting Enzyme Inhibitors

It is well known that angiotensin-converting enzyme inhibitors (ACE-I) are associated with the occurrence of angioedema in about 0.7% of individuals who receive this medication.[11,12] It has been reported that ACE-I can induce an exacerbation of symptoms in patients with HAE-C1-INH.[13] A 60-year-old man from a family with HAEnCI was reported who has had arterial hypertension since age 30 and had 4 tongue swellings following treatments with captopril and enalapril.[14] The last episode occurred when the patient received only hydrochlorothiazide and metoprolol. The patient has had no other symptoms of HAE. Two further patients with an exacerbation of HAEnCI after commencing ACE-I intake have been reported.[7] These observations demonstrate that ACE-I might have a trigger function with regard to HAEnCI. HAEnCI shares this feature with HAE-C1-INH. This state of affairs points to an important role of bradykinin in the pathogenesis of HAEnCI.

Angiotensin II Type 1 Receptor Antagonists

Two unrelated patients with preexisting HAEnCI were described who experienced severe exacerbation of symptoms associated with using angiotensin II type 1 receptor

Table 2
Influence of OC, pregnancies, and HRT on HAE-FXII in 35 women

	Intake of OC, n (%)	Pregnancy, n (%)	Receiving HRT, n (%)
Induction of the first clinical symptoms of HAE-FXII	17 (63.0)	3 (12)	0 (0)
Exacerbation of the preexisting symptomatic HAE-FXII	8 (29.6)	7 (28)	3 (42.9)
No influence	2 (7.4)	10 (40)	4 (57.1)
Improvement of symptoms	0 (0)	5 (20)	0 (0)
Total	27 (100)	25 (100)	7 (100)

Data from Bork K, Wulff K, Hardt J, et al. Hereditary angioedema caused by missense mutations in the factor XII gene: clinical features, trigger factors, and therapy. J Allergy Clin Immunol 2009;124:129–34.

antagonists (ARB).[15] A possible pathogenetic relationship between the underlying disease and the drug-associated angioedema was suggested.

GENDER

The disease has been observed predominantly in women.[1–3,5,8,9] In 2 families, however, the existence of clinically unaffected male carriers has been deduced.[2,3] In 2006 a family with dominantly inherited angioedema and normal C1 inhibitor was described in which not only 5 female but also 3 male family members were clinically affected.[14] Later additional male patients with HAEnCI were reported, among them also patients with HAE-FXII.[8,16,17]

INHERITANCE

Within the 43 families described in 2007,[8] between 2 and 10 members per family were affected. The examination of the pedigrees of the 43 families revealed that 2 successive generations were affected in 30 families, 3 successive generations were affected in 9 families, and 4 successive generations were affected in 4 families. These results support the assumption that HAEnCI is autosomally inherited with incomplete phenotypical penetrance.[1] An autosomal-dominant inheritance was also shown in HAE-FXII.[7]

GENETIC RESULTS

In 2001 the author of this article initiated a microsatellite scan of the total genome (performed by Dr C. Hennies, Max-Delbrück Center, Berlin) in 4 HAEnCI families that revealed major linkage signals for chromosomes 6 and 16 but not for chromosome 5 (Hennies C, personal communication, 2003). By following a functional hypothesis that the genetic defect might be located in the gene encoding the coagulation factor XII (F12) gene, the *F12* gene on chromosome 5 was then selectively investigated.[5] In May 2006, genetic mutations in 6 index patients of 20 families and in 22 patients of the corresponding 6 families were identified: 2 different missense mutations have been verified that were assumed to be responsible for the disease according to the cosegregation pattern.[5] The location of these mutations is the same locus, 5q33-qter of the Hageman factor or coagulation FXII gene (Online Mendelian Inheritance in Man no. 610619). Both mutations are located in exactly the same position, namely, in the second position of the codon (ACG) encoding amino acid residue 328 (or, if the leader peptide of FXII is not included in the numbering of amino acids, 309) of the mature protein, a threonine residue. One mutation leads to a threonine-to-lysine substitution (p.Thr328Lys), and the other to a threonine-to-arginine substitution (p.Thr328Arg). The mutations were located on exon 9. It was also found that the index patients of 14 further families with HAE and normal C1-INH did not show these mutations.[5] In accordance with the dominant inheritance pattern of the disease, patients were heterozygous for the respective mutations. Neither of the 2 mutations was detected in 145 healthy control individuals in this control panel. In 6 of the 20 families, 20 individuals, all female, were clinically diagnosed with HAEnCI. All these 20 women were found to be heterozygous carriers of either the Thr328Lys or the Thr328Arg mutation. Two additional women carried the Thr328Lys mutation but have not experienced any angioedema symptoms until now. Finally, there were 8 male heterozygous carriers of a missense mutation of Thr328, all symptom-free.[5]

Until now, the Thr328Lys mutation has been reported in numerous families (see **Box 2**).[5,7,16–27] The Thr328Arg mutation has been described only twice, both families coming from the patient series of Mainz.[5,7]

In 2011, a novel mutation, the deletion of 72 base pairs (c.971_1018+24del72), was identified in 3 members of a family originating from Turkey. The family included 2 sisters having HAEnCI and their symptom-free father displaying the same mutation (**Fig. 1**). The deletion started at c.971A (coding p.Lys324) in exon 9 and finished 24 base pairs downstream of intron 9. In the mutant *F12* alleles, the authentic donor splice site of exon 9 was deleted. The *F12* gene deletion was located in the gene region coding the proline-rich region of the FXII protein, which comprises the amino acids 315 to 368.

The novel mutation (ie, the deletion of c.971_1018+24del72) was heterozygous in the *F12* gene of the 2 sisters and their symptom-free father. All other members of this family were symptom-free and did not have the *F12* deletion. Three *F12* gene

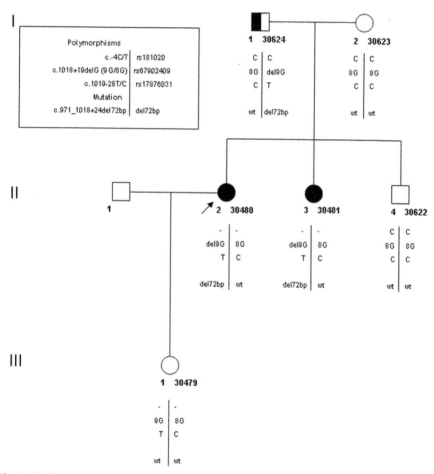

Fig. 1. Pedigree of a family with hereditary angioedema with normal C1-inhibitor. Results of the *F12* mutation analysis and the haplotypes using three *F12* gene polymorphisms are presented. Filled symbols, heterozygous deletion carrier with symptoms of angioedema; half-filled symbol, symptom-free heterozygous deletion carrier; unfilled symbols, symptom-free, without the *F12* deletion. (*Data from* Bork K, Wulff K, Meinke P, et al. A novel mutation in the coagulation factor 12 gene in subjects with hereditary angioedema and normal C1-inhibitor. Clin Immunol 2011;141:31–5.)

polymorphisms were used for haplotyping of the mutant alleles (see **Fig. 1**). The DNA region of the polymorphism c.1018+18delG (rs67902409) in intron 9 was involved in the deletion. As expected, the haplotype of the novel *F12* deletion allele was different from the haplotype of the well-known HAE-FXII allele p.Lys328.[5,18]

The deletion of c.971_1018+24del72 was not present in the 183 control subjects (366 independent chromosomes) comprising 84 male and 99 female subjects.

In **Fig. 2**, the FXII protein domains are presented with localization of the novel and the previously described *F12* gene mutations in the proline-rich region.

C1-INH activity and C4 in plasma were normal in most patients and slightly decreased in a small proportion of patients.[7,8,17,26] Therefore, right from the beginning, in the year 2000, it seemed to be improbable that the cause of the disease would be a mutation in the C1-INH gene. Binkley and Davis[2] found no abnormalities in either the 5′ regulatory region or the coding sequences of the C1-INH gene in affected individuals.

In most families with HAEnCl patients, a mutation in the *F12* gene could not be found. The author proposed the name "HAE-unknown" for this variant of disease.[7]

POTENTIAL ROLE OF THE MUTATIONS IN THE *F12* GENE IN HAE-FXII

The predicted structural and functional impact of the mutations in the *F12* gene, their absence in healthy controls, and their co-segregation with the phenotype in women provide strong support for the idea that these mutations cause disease. The remarkable observations that (1) 3 different mutations seen in patients but not controls; they affect the identical DNA position, and (2) all 3 lead to substitution of the wild-type threonine residue by a positively charged residue, lend further support to the assumption that these mutations play a disease-causing role.

It is not clear how the mutations in the *F12* gene could cause HAE-FXII (ie, the tendency to develop recurrent and self-limiting edema attacks in various organs). There are several arguments for the assumption that the KKS, also known as the "contact system" or "contact activation system," might be involved in the pathogenesis: (1) the causative mutations are in the FXII gene, and FXII is part of KKS; (2) KKS activation with the release of bradykinin at the end of the cascade is known to cause the acute attacks of HAE-C1-INH; (3) icatibant, a bradykinin B2 receptor antagonist, is effective in acute attacks of HAEnCl; and (4) corticosteroids and antihistamines are therapeutically ineffective for the treatment of swelling in HAE-FXII; therefore, histamine does not seem to play a major role in HAE-FXII.

Coagulation factor XII is a serine protease circulating in human plasma as a single-chain inactive zymogen at a concentration of approximately 30 μg/mL.[28–31] On contact with negatively charged surfaces, factor XII is activated by autoactivation and by plasma kallikrein, which itself is generated from prekallikrein by activated factor XII, high-molecular weight kininogen serving as a cofactor for reciprocal activation of factor XII, and prekallikrein. Factor XII, prekallikrein and high molecular weight kininogen form the KKS or "contact" system. Factor XII can be activated by negatively charged surfaces. In addition factor XII can be activated by activated factor XII (autoactivation). Prekallikrein can be activated to kallikrein by activated factor XII and/or cell-released proteases. Kallikrein splits bradykinin from high molecular weight kininogen. Activated factor XII and kallikrein are inactivated by C1 inhibitor. Factor XII is a typical mosaic protein: following a leader peptide of 19 residues, the mature plasma protein consists of 596 amino acids and is organized in an N-terminal fibronectin type II domain, followed by an epidermal growth factor-like domain, a fibronectin type-I domain, another epidermal growth factor-like domain, a kringle domain, a proline-rich region, and the C-terminal catalytic serine protease domain.[30]

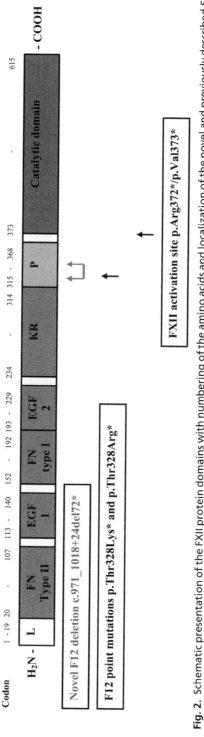

Fig. 2. Schematic presentation of the FXII protein domains with numbering of the amino acids and localization of the novel and previously described *F12* gene mutations in the proline-rich region that differs in HAE-FXII patients (*arrows*). EGF 1 or EGF 2, epidermal growth factor-like 1 or 2 domain; FN type I or FN type II, fibronectin type I or II domain; KR, kringle domain; L, signal or leader peptide; P, proline-rich region; * identify new numbering according to Ensembl. (*Data from* Bork K, Wulff K, Meinke P, et al. A novel mutation in the coagulation factor 12 gene in subjects with hereditary angioedema and normal C1-inhibitor. Clin Immunol 2011;141:31–5.)

The described amino acid substitutions are located in the poorly characterized proline-rich region of factor XII.[5,6] This region seems to play some role in the binding of factor XII to negatively charged surfaces.[31,32] Thus, one may speculate that those mutations may influence mechanisms of contact activation and may eventually inappropriately facilitate factor XII activation.

A report of patients with HAE-FXII demonstrated a more than 4-fold increase in FXIIa amidolytic activity on S-2302 compared with healthy controls.[18] The increased enzymatic activity was blocked completely by 2 mM PCK, and the report stated that PCK specifically inhibits FXII activation in human plasma. Based on these findings, it was suggested that the FXII Thr328Lys mutation is a gain-of-function mutation that markedly increases FXII amidolytic activity but that does not alter FXII plasma levels.[18] In a more recent study, elements of the KKS and the downstream-linked coagulation, complement, and fibrinolytic systems in the plasma of 6 patients with HAE-FXII with the Thr328Lys mutation and healthy probands were examined.[33] The mean FXII clotting activity was 90% in patients with the *F12* gene mutation and the concentration of FXIIa was 4.1 ng/mL; this did not differ from healthy probands. Mean prekallikrein amidolytic activity and high molecular weight kininogen clotting activity were 130% and 144%, respectively, both higher than in healthy probands. The mean kallikrein-like activity of the HAE-FXII patients was 11.4 U/L and did not differ from the healthy probands. There was no difference in FXII surface activation by silicon dioxide or in kallikrein-like activity with and without activation by dextran sulfate. Contrary to the results of the study mentioned earlier,[18] no indication that the Thr328Lys mutation causes a "gain-of-function" of FXIIa was observed in this investigation. Hence, the functional role of the observed FXII gene mutations in HAE-FXII still remains unclear.

The mediator responsible for edema formation in HAEnCI is not known. However, consider the following facts: (1) there are many similarities concerning clinical symptoms of HAE-C1-INH and HAEnCI; (2) in both conditions there is a high percentage of women whose disease is negatively affected by estrogen-containing medications; (3) ACE-I may lead to an increase in frequency and severity of attacks in HAEnCI similar to HAE-C1-INH (HAE type I and II); and (4) the response to antihistamines and corticosteroids is lacking, at least in the patients reported up until now. These facts permit the speculation that edema formation in HAEnCI may also be related to the kinin pathway. It is possible that bradykinin is the most important mediator in HAEnCI, similar to HAE type I and II. This possibility is supported by the efficacy of treatment of HAEnCI attacks with icatibant, a bradykinin B2 receptor antagonist.

DIAGNOSIS

Up until now the clinical diagnosis of HAEnCI has required that patients have the above-mentioned clinical symptoms, one or more family members also affected with these symptoms, the exclusion of familial and hereditary chronic urticaria with urticaria-associated angioedema, and normal C1-INH activity and protein in plasma. The diagnosis "hereditary angioedema with coagulation factor XII gene mutation" (HAE-FXII) requires the corresponding demonstration of the mutation. Until now there was no further laboratory test that could confirm the diagnosis "HAEnCI."

The question of whether there are sporadic, nonfamilial cases cannot be answered satisfyingly today. For HAE-FXII, a few patients with no further affected family members have been reported.[17] It is not possible to identify sporadic cases of HAE without mutations in the *F12* gene (HAE-unknown) at present because there are no laboratory tests available to confirm the diagnosis of this subtype of HAEnCI.

DIFFERENTIAL DIAGNOSIS

The most important differential diagnosis of HAEnCI is the other types of recurrent angioedema. Angioedema is a clinical sign that belongs to various clinical entities. Some of them are due to a hereditary or acquired C1-INH deficiency such as HAE types I and II and acquired angioedema due to C1-INH deficiency. Other types are not associated with a C1-INH deficiency. Other than HAEnCI, they include angioedema due to ACE-I and ARB, angioedema associated with an urticaria, allergic or nonallergic angioedema caused by insect stings, food, drugs other than ACE-I and ARB, or certain diseases, and idiopathic angioedema.

MANAGEMENT
Treatment of Acute Attacks

Until now, acute angioedema attacks of HAEnCI were treated with a C1-INH concentrate, icatibant, tranexamic acid, corticosteroids, and antihistamines. In one study, 7 patients with HAE-FXII received a C1-INH concentrate (Berinert, CSL Behring Inc, Marburg, Germany) for 63 angioedema attacks.[7] One patient who received this agent once for an abdominal attack reported that it was not effective. In the other 6 patients, the agent was very or moderately effective. Several patients with HAEnCI were reported who were treated with icatibant, a bradykinin B2 receptor antagonist used for acute attacks of HAE-C1-INH.[17,34,35] Time to resolution of symptoms was 1 hour to 6 days. In one attack the symptoms recurred after 6 hours and necessitated a second injection of icatibant. Tranexamic acid was also used for the treatment of acute attacks.[17] Time to first resolution of symptoms ranged from 3 hours to 5 days.

In numerous patients with HAEnCI, angioedema attacks had been treated with corticosteroids and antihistamines (at a dosage of 100–250 mg once or more times daily); however, this treatment was ineffective in all cases.[1,7,36,37]

Prophylactic Treatment

Progesterone, danazol, and tranexamic acid have been used prophylactically to prevent angioedema attacks.[7] In one study, 8 patients with HAE-FXII received a progesterone-containing and estrogen-free OC.[7] Seven of these patients took desogestrel, which is a progestagen, for 1 to 6 years, for a total of 27 years. One of these 7 patients was switched to an implant with etonogestrel for 3 years. The remaining woman received injections of medroxyprogesterone for 3 years. The 8 women were symptom-free during progesterone treatment. One woman with HAE-FXII received danazol (200 mg), an attenuated androgen, daily for 12 years.[7] While on treatment, she was symptom-free. During these 12 years, she discontinued danazol twice. Each cessation of treatment was followed by a series of severe abdominal attacks, tongue swellings, and skin swellings, and each time the patient resumed treatment. To date, the patient has had no side effects from danazol treatment. A second patient who received danazol (100 mg) daily for 6 years for severe HAE symptoms was also free of symptoms during treatment. The dose was subsequently tapered and discontinued; during the 2 years between discontinuation and the present, no HAE symptoms were observed.[7] Other studies[3,37,38] have also shown an improvement in symptoms in patients with HAEnCI during treatment with danazol. One woman with HAE-FXII who started tranexamic acid therapy (4 g/d) has had no attacks with this treatment regimen.[7] Tranexamic acid was effective or partly effective in long-term prophylaxis in pregnancies.[17]

SUMMARY

Hereditary angioedema with normal C1 inhibitor (HAE type III) is clinically character-ized by recurrent angioedema affecting the skin, gastrointestinal tract, and larynx. Skin swellings are the most frequent symptoms of HAEnCl. Most often they occur on the face, less frequently at the extremities, and only in rare cases at the genitals. Tongue swellings and abdominal pain attacks are less frequent symptoms. Laryngeal edema is rare. Death by asphyxiation as a result of attacks of upper airway obstruction has been observed. Women are more often affected than men. In some women the clinical symptoms of HAEnCl occur exclusively in periods of OC, HRT, or pregnancies, indicating that estrogens may have a considerable influence on the phenotypical dis-ease expression. Only limited data on the molecular basis of HAEnCl are currently available. In some families with HAEnCl, mutations in the FXII gene have been found in the affected patients. The co-segregation of these mutations with the disease phenotype demonstrates the causative role of the mutations. Several treatment op-tions are available for HAEnCl, including C1-INH agents, icatibant, progesterone, da-nazol, and tranexamic acid.

REFERENCES

1. Bork K, Barnstedt SE, Koch P, et al. Hereditary angioedema with normal C1-inhibitor activity in women. Lancet 2000;356:213–7.
2. Binkley KE, Davis A 3rd. Clinical, biochemical, and genetic characterization of a novel estrogen-dependent inherited form of angioedema. J Allergy Clin Immunol 2000;106:546–50.
3. Martin L, Degenne D, Toutain A, et al. Hereditary angioedema type III: an addi-tional French pedigree with autosomal dominant transmission. J Allergy Clin Im-munol 2001;107:747–8.
4. Zuraw BL, Bork K, Binkley KE, et al. Hereditary angioedema with normal C1 inhib-itor function: consensus of an international expert panel. Allergy Asthma Proc 2012;33(Suppl 1):S145–56.
5. Dewald G, Bork K. Missense mutations in the coagulation factor XII (Hageman factor) gene in hereditary angioedema with normal C1 inhibitor. Biochem Biophys Res Commun 2006;343:1286–9.
6. Bork K, Wulff K, Meinke P, et al. A novel mutation in the coagulation factor 12 gene in subjects with hereditary angioedema and normal C1-inhibitor. Clin Immunol 2011;141:31–5.
7. Bork K, Wulff K, Hardt J, et al. Hereditary angioedema caused by missense mutations in the factor XII gene: clinical features, trigger factors, and therapy. J Allergy Clin Immunol 2009;124:129–34.
8. Bork K, Gul D, Hardt J, et al. Hereditary angioedema with normal C1 inhibitor: clinical symptoms and course. Am J Med 2007;120:987–92.
9. Bork K, Fischer B, Dewald G. Recurrent episodes of skin angioedema and severe attacks of abdominal pain induced by oral contraceptives or hormone replace-ment therapy. Am J Med 2003;114:294–8.
10. Binkley KE, Davis AE 3rd. Estrogen-dependent inherited angioedema. Transfus Apher Sci 2003;29:215–9.
11. Sabroe RA, Black AK. Angiotensin-converting enzyme (ACE) inhibitors and angio-oedema. Br J Dermatol 1997;136:153–8.
12. Vleeming W, van Amsterdam JG, Stricker BH, et al. ACE inhibitor-induced an-gioedema. Incidence, prevention and management. Drug Saf 1998;18:171–88.

13. Agostoni A, Cicardi M. Contraindications to the use of ace inhibitors in patients with C1 esterase inhibitor deficiency. Am J Med 1991;90:278.
14. Bork K, Gul D, Dewald G. Hereditary angio-oedema with normal C1 inhibitor in a family with affected women and men. Br J Dermatol 2006;154:542–5.
15. Bork K, Dewald G. Hereditary angioedema type III, angioedema associated with angiotensin II receptor antagonists, and female sex. Am J Med 2004;116:644–5.
16. Martin L, Raison-Peyron N, Nothen MM, et al. Hereditary angioedema with normal C1 inhibitor gene in a family with affected women and men is associated with the p.Thr328Lys mutation in the F12 gene. J Allergy Clin Immunol 2007;120:975–7.
17. Marcos C, Lopez Lera A, Varela S, et al. Clinical, biochemical, and genetic characterization of type III hereditary angioedema in 13 Northwest Spanish families. Ann Allergy Asthma Immunol 2012;109:195–200.e2.
18. Cichon S, Martin L, Hennies HC, et al. Increased activity of coagulation factor XII (Hageman factor) causes hereditary angioedema type III. Am J Hum Genet 2006;79:1098–104.
19. Bouillet L, Ponard D, Rousset H, et al. A case of hereditary angio-oedema type III presenting with C1-inhibitor cleavage and a missense mutation in the F12 gene. Br J Dermatol 2007;156:1063–5.
20. Bell CG, Kwan E, Nolan RC, et al. First molecular confirmation of an Australian case of type III hereditary angioedema. Pathology 2008;40:82–3.
21. Prieto A, Tornero P, Rubio M, et al. Missense mutation Thr309Lys in the coagulation factor XII gene in a Spanish family with hereditary angioedema type III. Allergy 2009;64:284–6.
22. Duan QL, Binkley K, Rouleau GA. Genetic analysis of Factor XII and bradykinin catabolic enzymes in a family with estrogen-dependent inherited angioedema. J Allergy Clin Immunol 2009;123:906–10.
23. Nagy N, Greaves MW, Tanaka A, et al. Recurrent European missense mutation in the F12 gene in a British family with type III hereditary angioedema. J Dermatol Sci 2009;56:62–4.
24. Hentges F, Hilger C, Kohnen M, et al. Angioedema and estrogen-dependent angioedema with activation of the contact system. J Allergy Clin Immunol 2009;123:262–4.
25. Picone O, Donnadieu AC, Brivet FG, et al. Obstetrical complications and outcome in two families with hereditary angioedema due to mutation in the F12 gene. Obstet Gynecol Int 2010;2010:957507.
26. Vitrat-Hincky V, Gompel A, Dumestre-Perard C, et al. Type III hereditary angio-oedema: clinical and biological features in a French cohort. Allergy 2010;65:1331–6.
27. Baeza ML, Rodriguez-Marco A, Prieto A, et al. Factor XII gene missense mutation Thr328Lys in an Arab family with hereditary angioedema type III. Allergy 2011;66:981–2.
28. Kaplan AP, Joseph K, Shibayama Y, et al. The intrinsic coagulation/kinin-forming cascade: assembly in plasma and cell surfaces in inflammation. Adv Immunol 1997;66:225–72.
29. Cool DE, MacGillivray RT. Characterization of the human blood coagulation factor XII gene. Intron/exon gene organization and analysis of the 5'-flanking region. J Biol Chem 1987;262:13662–73.
30. Cool DE, Edgell CJ, Loule GV, et al. Characterization of human blood coagulation factor XII cDNA. Prediction of the primary structure of factor XII and the tertiary structure of beta-factor XIIa. J Biol Chem 1985;260:13666–76.

31. Citarella F, Aiuti A, La Porta C, et al. Control of human coagulation by recombinant serine proteases. Blood clotting is activated by recombinant factor XII deleted of five regulatory domains. Eur J Biochem 1992;208:23–30.

32. Citarella F, Ravon DM, Pascucci B, et al. Structure/function analysis of human factor XII using recombinant deletion mutants. Evidence for an additional region involved in the binding to negatively charged surfaces. Eur J Biochem 1996; 238:240–9.

33. Bork K, Kleist R, Hardt J, et al. Kallikrein-kinin system and fibrinolysis in hereditary angioedema due to the factor XII gene mutation Thr309Lys. Blood Coagul Fibrinolysis 2009;20:325–32.

34. Bouillet L, Boccon-Gibod I, Ponard D, et al. Bradykinin receptor 2 antagonist (icatibant) for hereditary angioedema type III attacks. Ann Allergy Asthma Immunol 2009;103:448.

35. Boccon-Gibod I, Bouillet L. Safety and efficacy of icatibant self-administration for acute hereditary angioedema. Clin Exp Immunol 2012;168:303–7.

36. Serrano C, Guilarte M, Tella R, et al. Oestrogen-dependent hereditary angio-oedema with normal C1 inhibitor: description of six new cases and review of pathogenic mechanisms and treatment. Allergy 2008;63:735–41.

37. Herrmann G, Schneider L, Krieg T, et al. Efficacy of danazol treatment in a patient with the new variant of hereditary angio-oedema (HAE III). Br J Dermatol 2004; 150:157–8.

38. Bork K. Hereditary angioedema with normal C1 inhibitor activity including hereditary angioedema with coagulation factor XII gene mutations. Immunol Allergy Clin North Am 2006;26:709–24.

Creating a Comprehensive Treatment Plan for Hereditary Angioedema

Marc A. Riedl, MD, MS

KEYWORDS

- Hereditary angioedema • C1INH deficiency • Therapy • Treatment plan

KEY POINTS

- Management of hereditary angioedema (HAE) has become increasingly complex with the recent clinical development of additional therapies.
- A comprehensive HAE treatment plan aims to prevent mortality, minimize disability, and significantly improve patients' quality of life.
- Important components of the HAE treatment plan include patient education, reliable access to effective HAE-specific medications, and consistent follow-up to monitor therapeutic efficacy and safety.
- A rapid, reliable acute treatment plan is essential for every HAE patient without exception; long-term prophylaxis may confer additional benefit in select patients.
- Early treatment of HAE attacks reduces the duration of angioedema episodes; self-administration or home health programs may facilitate rapid treatment.

INTRODUCTION

Hereditary angioedema (HAE) is a rare genetic condition causing unpredictable intermittent episodes of cutaneous or mucosal tissue swelling.[1] Three subtypes of HAE have been identified: HAE due to quantitative deficiency of C1-esterase inhibitor (C1INH) protein (Type I), HAE due to functional deficiency of C1INH (Type II), and HAE with normal C1INH due to a heretofore undetermined biochemical cause, but sometimes associated with Factor XII mutations (Type III).[2–4] All subtypes of HAE manifest with angioedema episodes commonly involving 3 anatomic sites: (1) skin/subcutaneous tissues including the extremities, face, and genitalia; (2) the gastrointestinal tract; and (3) the upper airway including oropharynx and larynx. Swelling episodes typically last 2 to 5 days and are often debilitating because of pain, disfigurement,

Division of Rheumatology, Allergy and Immunology, University of California - San Diego, 9500 Gilman Dr., La Jolla, CA 92093, USA
E-mail addresses: mriedl@mednet.ucla.edu; mriedl@ucsd.edu

Immunol Allergy Clin N Am 33 (2013) 471–485
http://dx.doi.org/10.1016/j.iac.2013.07.003
0889-8561/13/$ – see front matter © 2013 Elsevier Inc. All rights reserved.

and loss of functional capacity. Attacks involving the upper airway are life-threatening, owing to the risk of asphyxiation. HAE swelling of the upper airway continues to cause fatalities despite the availability of effective therapies.[5] Because of the substantial disability and mortality associated with HAE, implementation of an effective management plan for every patient is critical. This article outlines important considerations in developing and optimizing the treatment of individuals affected by HAE.

In this context it is worth noting that HAE is frequently undiagnosed or misdiagnosed. Multiple studies have documented the diagnostic delay experienced by many affected patients, with a median time of 13 to 22 years from first symptoms to diagnosis.[6–8] Thus, HAE must be considered in the differential diagnosis of recurring angioedema such that appropriate laboratory testing can be conducted to confirm or exclude the condition. The importance of properly diagnosing the cause of angioedema is highlighted by the fact that antihistamines and corticosteroids, useful for treating more common allergic or histamine-mediated forms of angioedema, are entirely ineffective in treating HAE.[9] Detailed pathophysiology is not covered here, but angioedema associated with HAE is due to dysregulation of the kallikrein-bradykinin system.[10] Effective HAE treatment therefore requires therapy that targets this pathway.

GENERAL HAE TREATMENT CONCEPTS, CONSENSUS DOCUMENTS, AND SPECIALIST CARE

Broadly, HAE therapy can be divided into acute (on-demand) treatment administered at the onset of angioedema symptoms, and prophylactic treatment given when a patient is asymptomatic to prevent angioedema from occurring.[11] Prophylactic therapy can be further subdivided into long-term (or routine) prophylaxis given regularly over extended periods of time (months to years) to reduce frequency and severity of attacks, and short-term prophylaxis typically given for brief periods (days) to prevent swelling during a specific event (ie, surgical or dental procedure). The management of HAE has rapidly evolved in recent years through robust translational and clinical research efforts, resulting in the availability of newly licensed therapies for HAE.[12] With these advances, several expert groups have published consensus recommendations intended to provide guidance for the clinical care of HAE patients.[13–16] In presenting the major components of an HAE management plan, these publications should be recognized as important references for clinicians managing HAE patients. Existing evidence-based consensus publications generally agree on the following HAE management principles:

1. On-demand treatment with an effective HAE-specific medication must be available for every HAE patient, including those on prophylactic therapy. This on-demand medication should be reliably and efficiently accessible.
2. All or nearly all HAE angioedema episodes are eligible for treatment.
3. Airway angioedema is uniquely life threatening and requires special attention.
4. Early treatment of HAE attacks is beneficial in reducing morbidity and complications.
5. Prophylactic treatment is indicated for patients in whom on-demand treatment alone is unsatisfactory.

These areas of broad consensus are central to developing effective HAE treatment plans. In addition, consensus documents generally recommend "HAE specialist" involvement in the medical care of patients affected by this condition. Given the rarity, complexity, and severity of HAE, it is generally recognized that patients benefit from consultation with health care providers (HCPs) possessing expertise and clinical experience in HAE treatment. Owing to the specialized nature of HAE care, large referral centers exist in some countries to provide nationwide patient access to the most comprehensive evaluation and treatment.[17–20] Development of management plans and periodic evaluation occur at the center, while coordination with local physicians is necessary to implement the details of therapy and provide ongoing support.

PATIENT EDUCATION AND COUNSELING

A comprehensive management plan for HAE patients includes numerous components (**Box 1**). Although prescribing and administering medication is essential for optimal management of HAE, the first step in implementing effective treatment is to provide condition-specific education for patients and their family. Patients and/or caregivers who have a basic understanding of the symptoms, natural course of angioedema episodes, and potential complications of HAE more readily achieve rational and effective use of HAE medications. A tactful but clear explanation of the substantial risk of asphyxiation with airway swelling is important, with emphasis on the requirement for rapid medical evaluation during such attacks, even when effective on-demand treatment has been administered. Many HAE patients have experienced numerous attacks and are well versed in the clinical manifestations and patterns of their episodes. However, because of the tremendous clinical variability of HAE, other patients may have less experience with symptoms and may not readily recognize early signs or potential complications associated with skin, gastrointestinal, and/or airway swelling.

The clinical course of HAE is unpredictable; patients and families should understand the potential for any type of angioedema attack at any time. Many patients also experience prodromal symptoms that precede angioedema episodes.[21] Although prodromal symptoms are at times nonspecific, awareness of these may be helpful in rapidly identifying evolving episodes, thereby leading to earlier treatment if and when swelling ensues. Families should be informed of the hereditary nature of this autosomal dominant condition. It is generally advisable for first-degree relatives of HAE patients to be screened for the condition, although this is a personal decision to be discussed with each individual and the HAE specialist.

Recognition of attack triggers is an additional important educational component. Although variable from patient to patient, several specific factors are known to exacerbate HAE swelling episodes in a large percentage of patients.[22] Some triggers are avoidable, including medications such as angiotensin-converting enzyme inhibitors and estrogen therapies. Others can be actively managed, such as the iatrogenic trauma of surgical or dental procedures when short-term prophylactic medications can be administered to reduce angioedema risk. Some trigger factors are less "modifiable": incidental trauma, acute infection, and psychological stress are all recognized to increase the frequency of HAE attacks in some patients. However, patients' awareness of these factors may improve their understanding of exacerbating events and enable preparation or factor modification when possible.

The initial discussion about HAE should ultimately seek to assess the impact of the condition on the individual's quality of life. HAE-specific quality-of-life measurement tools have only recently been developed.[23] However, it is useful to evaluate the impact of HAE symptoms on the patient's work, school, family, and social activities. Patients may have anxiety or depression related to chronic illness, or resulting from traumatic personal HAE-related events (eg, intubation/tracheostomy or HAE fatality in the family).[24] For some patients, a comprehensive treatment plan may include

> ## Box 1
> ### Suggested steps in developing a comprehensive HAE treatment plan
>
> *Initial Evaluation of Confirmed HAE*
> - Assess current features of angioedema (frequency, severity, anatomic location, treatment, impact on activities/quality of life)
> - Educate patient and family on HAE symptoms, triggers, prodromes, risks, genetics, screening
> - Discuss treatment goals for patient
> - Discuss required acute treatment plan, comparative medication options
> - Discuss option of routine prophylaxis, comparative medication options
> - Discuss benefits of early acute treatment
> - Discuss unique risks of airway angioedema warranting medical evaluation
> - Discuss indications for short-term prophylaxis (surgical, medical, or dental procedures)
>
> *Following Selection of Therapeutic Agent(s)*
> - Determine if candidate for self-administration based on patient and medication factors
> - Determine site of treatment (self-administration vs home health provider vs medical facility)
> - Provide patient-specific prescription and clinical documentation for processing/payor authorization
> - Arrange self-administration training (in office or via home health) as applicable
> - Determine plan for reporting use of medication: scheduled office visit, phone, e-communication, home health reports
> - Determine plan for communication of treatment plan to local health care providers, integration of care as applicable
> - Provide tools for navigating health system: written treatment plan, letter, USB drive, medical alert bracelet
> - Provide resources for ongoing education
>
> *Periodic Follow-Up Evaluations*
> - Assess current features of angioedema (triggers, frequency, severity, anatomic location, treatment impact on activities/quality of life)
> - Review medication use: frequency and efficacy
> - Review medication adverse effects; safety laboratory tests if indicated (androgens: semiannual liver function tests, lipid profile, complete blood count, urinalysis, annual liver ultrasonography; plasma-derived C1INH: consider annual hepatitis B/C, human immunodeficiency virus testing)
> - Discuss obstacles to treatment; identify reasons for untreated symptoms that interfered with activity
> - Review interactions/communication with other health care providers; integration of care
> - Review whether patient goals are achieved with current treatment plan
> - Consider treatment adjustments if goals are not achieved (change acute medication or plan logistics, add/remove/titrate prophylactic therapy as clinically indicated)
> - Ensure medication refills are provided
> - Review benefits of early acute treatment
> - Review unique risks of airway angioedema
> - Review anticipated indications for short-term prophylaxis

psychological counseling to address these condition-related issues. The discussion may also elucidate specific treatment goals of the patient such as returning to the workforce, pursuing a degree or career, embarking on travel, or reducing side effects from current treatment. Such details can help to establish reasonable objective expectations for both patient and physician, and implement a management plan aimed at improving the quality of life.

Because of the complexity and volume of information that newly diagnosed HAE patients must assimilate, referral to durable educational materials is strongly recommended. Video segments, online educational programs, and handouts are useful in allowing patients to review and absorb information at their own pace. In addition, national and regional support programs are available for patients and families who are interested in connecting with other HAE patients. The United States Hereditary Angioedema Association (www.haea.org), a patient advocacy group, provides a variety of educational resources and services for individuals affected by HAE.

ACUTE TREATMENT

Every individual diagnosed with HAE requires an acute (on-demand) treatment plan,[13–16] given the unpredictable nature of angioedema attacks that may be rapidly life threatening, even in patients who historically have never experienced substantial HAE symptoms. Thus, the selection and prescribing of an effective acute medication for HAE is among the first priorities in managing the condition. Five medications (**Table 1**) have been rigorously studied for the treatment of HAE attacks, although country-specific licensing of these products varies. In the United States Berinert, Kalbitor, and Firazyr are approved for treating HAE attacks, whereas in Europe Berinert, Firazyr, Cinryze, and Ruconest are licensed for this indication. Based on clinical trial data and regulatory approvals, these medications can be regarded as generally safe and effective for the treatment of HAE attacks.[25–29] Direct comparisons of medication efficacy are not possible because of differences in study methodology and end point/outcome measures.[12] However, in developing management plans it is important that both physicians and patients understand basic differences between the medication options, such as variations in production source, route of administration, and safety/adverse-effect profiles. Physicians should be familiar with drug-specific considerations so as to provide guidance to patients on the potential risks and benefits of each medication. Patient-specific factors may also be important in selecting an acute therapy: examples include pregnancy, frequent travel, residence in a remote location, rapidity of angioedema progression, concomitant medical conditions, or previous adverse effects from a specific medication. Patients may express preference for a specific source (plasma vs synthetic), route (intravenous vs subcutaneous), or treatment model (self-administration vs home health vs health care facility). The physician-patient discussion should review both drug and patient factors, and ideally select the medication best suited to the patient's clinical situation and treatment preferences.

Once the acute treatment medication has been selected, access to the medication must be reliable and efficient, and this entails several steps:

1. Medication should be prescribed and provided for each individual patient. Because of the rarity of HAE, effective medications are not readily available in most hospitals or pharmacies. Patient-specific medication is required.
2. Prescriptions can be sent to centralized processing and authorization units supported by the specific pharmaceutical manufacturers. Owing to the cost of so-called orphan drugs, clinical documentation of the condition and a "letter of

Table 1
Specific medication options for the treatment of HAE

Medication and Manufacturer	FDA Approval Status	Approved Dose and Route	Mechanism of Action	Reported Side Effects
Acute (On-Demand) Medications				
Plasma-derived C1INH (Berinert), CSL Behring	Approved for acute attacks in adults and adolescents	20 U/kg intravenous	Inhibits plasma kallikrein, factors XIIa and XIa, C1s, C1r, plasmin	Rare: risk of anaphylaxis, thrombosis Theoretical: transmission of infectious agent
Recombinant human C1INH (Rhucin, Ruconest), Santarus/Sobi	Not approved; investigational drug for acute attacks	50 U/kg intravenous		Rare: risk of anaphylaxis
Ecallantide (Kalbitor), Dyax	Approved for acute attacks in ≥16 y age group	30 mg subcutaneous	Inhibits plasma kallikrein	Common: prolonged partial thromboplastin time Uncommon: risk of anaphylaxis (must be administered by health care professional)
Icatibant (Firazyr), Shire	Approved for acute attacks in ≥18 y age group	30 mg subcutaneous	Bradykinin-2 receptor antagonist	Common: local swelling, pain, pruritus at injection site Theoretical: worsening of an ongoing ischemic event

Prophylactic Medications

Plasma-derived C1INH (Cinryze), ViroPharma	Approved for routine prophylaxis of HAE attacks in adults and adolescents	1000 units every 3–4 d intravenously	Inhibits plasma kallikrein, factors XIIa and XIa, C1s, C1r, plasmin	Rare: risk of anaphylaxis, thrombosis; Theoretical: transmission of infectious agent
Danazol (Danacrine), Sanofi-Synthelabo	Approved for prophylaxis in adults	200 mg/d or less	17α-Alkylated androgen, mechanism unknown	Common: weight gain, virilization, acne, altered libido, muscle pain, headaches, depression, fatigue, nausea, constipation, menstrual abnormalities, increase in liver enzymes, hypertension, alterations in lipid profile; Uncommon: decreased growth rate in children, masculinization of female fetus, cholestatic jaundice, peliosis hepatis, hepatocellular adenoma
Stanozolol (Winstrol)	Approved for prophylaxis	2 mg/d or less		
Oxandralone (Oxandrin), Savient	Not approved	10 mg/d or less		
Methyltestosterone (Android), Valeant	Not approved	10 mg/d or less		

Abbreviation: FDA, US Food and Drug Administration.

necessity" are often required to obtain coverage for standard-of-care HAE medications.

3. Site of treatment must be determined (home vs health care facility) to direct medication shipment to the appropriate location. In general, 3 treatment models have been used: self-administration, home treatment via visiting nurse, and health care facility treatment (hospital, clinic, infusion center). Home treatment increasingly is preferred when safe and feasible, based on evidence that this treatment model reduces time to treatment and duration of swelling, and improves the quality of life.[30–32] It is usually beneficial for patients to have acute HAE medication in their possession so that it can be reliably accessed when needed. However, if the medication is taken to a hospital for administration, patients should check with the medical facility ahead of time to determine the acceptability of bringing in medication for dosing. Some hospitals and health care centers have policies prohibiting "brown-bagging" of patient medication. It is advisable for patients and HAE specialists to contact the medical center before an HAE emergency so that hospital officials and pharmacists are aware of the unique individualized treatment plan. Likewise, for patients with travel plans, self-administration or identification of available treatment sites before travel is prudent.

4. If self-administration of acute medication is elected, extensive patient instruction on proper techniques is critical. Training may be done in the physician's office or by various home nursing services. Berinert and Cinryze (Cinryze is licensed for acute HAE treatment in Europe) as well as Firazyr are approved for self-administration. Intravenous self-treatment requires more training in comparison with subcutaneous therapy, although many patients are capable of successfully performing either. Kalbitor is not approved for self-administration, but has effectively been administered by home health nurses. Home health services may be attractive to patients who prefer the presence of a HCP with the relative convenience of home treatment.

5. Patients should be advised that HAE acute medications generally take 30 to 60 minutes to begin relieving symptoms.[25–29] Patients benefit from treatment early in the attack so as to limit progression time and subsequent severity of angioedema symptoms.[30,33–35]

6. Although licensed HAE-specific acute medications are highly effective, clinical study data demonstrate that up to 30% of attacks require redosing because of refractory or recurrent symptoms, though most studies demonstrate a redosing rate of less than 15%.[25–39] Patients should be advised to keep at least 2 doses of acute medication available and be provided with directions on when to redose based on product-specific labeling and the HAE specialist's expertise.

7. All treatment plans should have a contingency plan for the patient in the event HAE therapy is ineffective or a complication such as an adverse drug reaction occurs. This plan may involve identifying the nearest hospital for evaluation, calling emergency services, and/or designating a family member or friend with knowledge of the patient's condition who is able to assist.

8. Acute treatment plans should include an information "feedback loop": the treating physician should be aware of events requiring medication use such that ongoing monitoring takes place and medication refills can be provided appropriately. This feedback may be transmitted remotely via phone/electronic communication, by scheduling periodic clinical visits, and by physician communication with the pharmacy and/or home health company servicing the patient. Ongoing evaluation is necessary to determine whether an acute treatment plan is achieving the treatment goals, and if not, how it may be improved.

PROPHYLACTIC TREATMENT

Long-term prophylactic therapy is not required in every patient with HAE. It is, however, an important consideration in many patients.[37] Given the dramatic variability of HAE symptoms in individuals over time, the author's practice is to discuss long-term prophylactic therapy options with every HAE patient at least briefly at their initial consultation, to ensure awareness of this treatment strategy if on-demand therapy alone is unsatisfactory at any point during their lifetime. Long-term prophylaxis may be initiated immediately in some newly diagnosed HAE patients based on disease severity and clinical circumstances; in other patients it may be added after a trial of on-demand therapy alone. No consensus criteria exist for the implementation of long-term prophylactic treatment in HAE.[14] Many HAE experts consider high frequency and severity of angioedema episodes to be the strongest indications for routine prophylaxis, but this strategy should be considered at any point when on-demand treatment alone is unsatisfactory; evidence is lacking to support any specific objective criteria.[38,39] The decision to institute or continue prophylactic treatment is made on an individual basis by the physician and patient with consideration of personal circumstances, disease course, and quality of life. Patients on routine prophylaxis still require an acute treatment plan, as "break-through" attacks occasionally occur on all forms of prophylactic therapy.[40,41]

Long-term prophylactic therapies are listed in **Table 1**. Based on efficacy data, attenuated androgens and plasma-derived C1INH are the recommended options for preventing HAE attacks.[13-16] Antifibrinolytics (tranexamic acid, aminocaproic acid) are recognized to have inferior efficacy data, and are now rarely recommended.[14,15] Because of the adverse effect profile and availability of other effective therapies, the use of androgens for HAE prophylaxis appears to have declined in some countries (Riedl MA, Banerji A and Gower R, personal communication, 2013).[18] Regardless of the prophylactic medication selected by the physician-patient team, the long-term nature of routine prophylactic treatment requires additional levels of monitoring to ensure both efficacy and safety. Of particular importance is regular assessment of liver function and lipid profiles in patients taking attenuated androgens.[42] Most consensus publications recommend daily dosing of less than 200 mg danazol or equivalent.[13-16] Monitoring of intravenous C1INH prophylaxis may include annual viral testing (hepatitis B and C, human immunodeficiency virus), given the repeated administration of a plasma product.[14] Thrombotic events with C1INH therapy are rare but reported, and peripheral venous access should be preserved as long as possible through careful infusion techniques.[43] Education in such techniques is particularly important for patients learning to self-infuse prophylactic C1INH. The placement of intravenous ports for routine C1INH infusions is inadvisable because of potential thrombotic and infectious complications. Occasionally peripheral vascular access is exhausted despite all precautions, and no alternative to port placement exists. However, in the opinion of the author, ports should be regarded as a last resort for C1INH infusions and the risks thoroughly discussed with the patient.

Interindividual and intraindividual response is variable with regard to effective doses of prophylactic medications.[40,44] Because no biomarker has been demonstrated to correlate with the efficacy of prophylactic therapies, clinical follow-up is the only method of determining whether a reduction in angioedema episodes is achieved. Dose adjustments of prophylactic medication, either increased or decreased, may be warranted over time commensurate with changes in HAE symptomatology. Thus, long-term prophylactic therapy is often not static but rather a dynamic process of reevaluation and adjustment to maximize efficacy and safety. Some patients require routine prophylaxis treatment for only discrete periods based on symptom fluctuation.

PREPARING THE PATIENT TO NAVIGATE THE HEALTH SYSTEM

HAE, as a rare condition, is unrecognized and unknown by many HCPs. As a result, HAE patients are frequently misdiagnosed and receive inappropriate and ineffective medical care, particularly in the acute care setting during an angioedema attack. At best this is frustrating; at worst it is harmful, as patients undergo unnecessary surgery for abdominal pain or receive ineffective medication for airway angioedema, leading to asphyxiation or emergency airway procedures. Thus, a major component of effective HAE management is equipping the patient to interact with HCPs who are not familiar with HAE. Recognizing that new effective therapies have allowed many patients to avoid emergency departments and hospitals for treatment, HAE patients still require medical evaluation for airway involvement on occasions when their treatment plan fails (ie, unsuccessful home treatment), and for other concomitant medical conditions.[45]

The HAE specialist plays an important role in communicating with other health care providers regarding care of the patient, which is particularly important in the setting of an HAE attack or during hospitalization when traumatic medical procedures may trigger angioedema symptoms.[46] Ideally, the patient or involved HCPs may reach the HAE specialist directly with questions and concerns. Brief letters and/or treatment action plans (**Fig. 1**) from the HAE specialist are useful in communicating the basic elements of effective HAE treatment to other HCPs, as well as serving as a helpful reference for the patient. These documents can be customized for the patient to include individualized medications and the HAE specialist's office contact information to facilitate further communication. It is recommended that patients have a letter, wallet card, and/or USB drive containing instructional files readily available in the event of emergency visits for angioedema. Medical-alert bracelets denoting HAE and required acute medication are advisable in the event a patient is incapacitated. Flagging of the electronic medical record at primary hospitals is another useful strategy that can prevent delays in effective treatment.

FOLLOW-UP AND MONITORING

After implementation of the initial treatment plan (acute therapy arrangements required, prophylactic therapy considered as appropriate), clinical follow-up should occur at regular intervals as determined by the HAE specialist. It is beneficial to speak with the patient following the initial use of any new medications to identify side effects or obstacles to effective treatment. Given the relative complexity of HAE treatment plans, the detailed logistics of medication use should be reviewed at each clinic visit: where is there medication stored, when is it being used, what is the treatment location, and who is administering the medication? This line of inquiry allows the patient and physician to identify any pitfalls and make adjustments. Occasionally a medication or treatment plan is not working well because of logistics or side effects, in which case wholesale changes may be necessary. Common issues for discussion and review at follow-up include which attacks are eligible to treat, when to initiate treatment, unique risks of airway events that require medical attention, development of any treatment-related side effects, and issues related to medication acquisition or refills. In the experience of the author, patients are at times reluctant to treat cutaneous attacks despite the functional impairment that develops, and also delay treatment until several hours into attacks when symptoms become severe, thus resulting in longer periods of disability. Ultimately the patient will determine when to use available

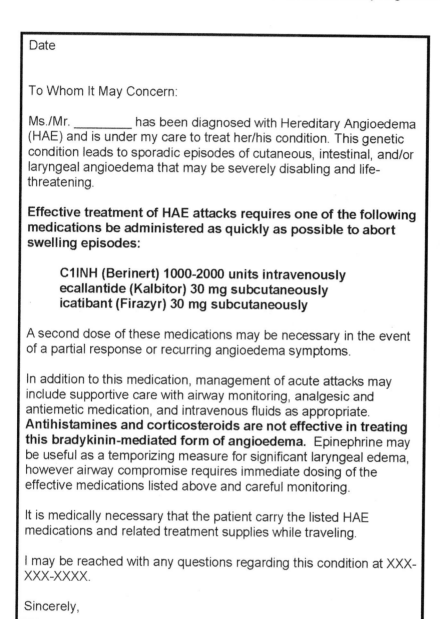

Date

To Whom It May Concern:

Ms./Mr. _____ has been diagnosed with Hereditary Angioedema (HAE) and is under my care to treat her/his condition. This genetic condition leads to sporadic episodes of cutaneous, intestinal, and/or laryngeal angioedema that may be severely disabling and life-threatening.

Effective treatment of HAE attacks requires one of the following medications be administered as quickly as possible to abort swelling episodes:

> **C1INH (Berinert) 1000-2000 units intravenously**
> **ecallantide (Kalbitor) 30 mg subcutaneously**
> **icatibant (Firazyr) 30 mg subcutaneously**

A second dose of these medications may be necessary in the event of a partial response or recurring angioedema symptoms.

In addition to this medication, management of acute attacks may include supportive care with airway monitoring, analgesic and antiemetic medication, and intravenous fluids as appropriate. **Antihistamines and corticosteroids are not effective in treating this bradykinin-mediated form of angioedema.** Epinephrine may be useful as a temporizing measure for significant laryngeal edema, however airway compromise requires immediate dosing of the effective medications listed above and careful monitoring.

It is medically necessary that the patient carry the listed HAE medications and related treatment supplies while traveling.

I may be reached with any questions regarding this condition at XXX-XXX-XXXX.

Sincerely,

Fig. 1. Sample letter and treatment action plan from the HAE specialist.

treatment, but the HAE specialist should regularly review with the patient the central management principles from published consensus guidelines, as these represent the current standard of care for HAE.

Box 2 lists suggested clinical data to be collected for each angioedema attack to fully evaluate these events at follow-up visits. Standardized tools to more comprehensively assess HAE disease activity and quality of life in the clinical setting are in development, but not yet widely used or validated.[23] Analogous to asthma evaluation tools, these may allow rapid identification of patients who are suboptimally managed and

---

Box 2
Suggested data collection on HAE attacks

Angioedema Attack Details

Date and time of symptom onset

Anatomic location of swelling

Prodromal symptoms experienced (if applicable)

Triggering event (if known)

Severity/degree of interference with activities

Attack Treatment Details

HAE-specific acute treatment used

Date and time treatment administered

Date and time symptoms began to improve

Date and time symptoms were completely resolved

Redosing of HAE-specific medication required

Adverse events associated with treatment

Obstacles to timely use of HAE-specific medication

Emergency department and/or hospitalization required

Treatment required in additional to HAE-specific medication (analgesics, antiemetics, and so forth)

---

may benefit from changes in treatment. Real-time clinical reports from patients via mobile devices may allow HAE specialists to more quickly respond to poorly managed HAE symptoms with revised treatment recommendations. Efforts are also ongoing to harmonize clinical data collection worldwide such that with patient consent, deidentified data could be compiled globally to analyze relatively large cohorts of patients treated in the real-world setting: an otherwise difficult task in rare medical conditions.[14] This approach may identify specific treatment models, practices, or variables that can improve clinical outcomes.

REFERENCES

1. Zuraw BL. Clinical practice. Hereditary angioedema. N Engl J Med 2008;359:1027–36.
2. Donaldson VH, Evans RR. A biochemical abnormality in hereditary angioneurotic edema: absence of serum inhibitor of C'1-esterase. Am J Med 1963;35:37–44.
3. Rosen FS, Pensky J, Donaldson V, et al. Hereditary angioneurotic edema: two genetic variants. Science 1965;148:957–8.
4. Bork K, Barnstedt SE, Koch P, et al. Hereditary angioedema with normal C1-inhibitor activity in women. Lancet 2000;356:213–7.
5. Bork K, Hardt J, Witzke G. Fatal laryngeal attacks and mortality in hereditary angioedema due to C1-INH deficiency. J Allergy Clin Immunol 2012;130:692–7.
6. Roche O, Blanch A, Caballero T, et al. Hereditary angioedema due to C1 inhibitor deficiency: patient registry and approach to the prevalence in Spain. Ann Allergy Asthma Immunol 2005;94(4):498–503.
7. Bygum A. Hereditary angio-oedema in Denmark: a nationwide survey. Br J Dermatol 2009;161(5):1153–8.

8. Frank MM, Gelfand JA, Atkinson JP. Hereditary angioedema: the clinical syndrome and its management. Ann Intern Med 1976;84(5):580–93.
9. Farkas H. Current pharmacotherapy of bradykinin-mediated angioedema. Expert Opin Pharmacother 2013;14(5):571–86.
10. Kaplan AP. Enzymatic pathways in the pathogenesis of hereditary angioedema: the role of C1 inhibitor therapy. J Allergy Clin Immunol 2010;126(5): 918–25.
11. Bork K, Davis-Lorton M. Overview of hereditary angioedema caused by C1-inhibitor deficiency: assessment and clinical management. Eur Ann Allergy Clin Immunol 2013;45(1):7–16.
12. Parikh N, Riedl MA. New therapeutics in C1INH deficiency: a review of recent studies and advances. Curr Allergy Asthma Rep 2011;11(4):300–8.
13. Bowen T, Cicardi M, Farkas H, et al. 2010 International consensus algorithm for the diagnosis, therapy and management of hereditary angioedema. Allergy Asthma Clin Immunol 2010;6:24.
14. Cicardi M, Bork K, Caballero T, et al. Evidence-based recommendations for the therapeutic management of angioedema owing to hereditary C1 inhibitor deficiency: consensus report of an International Working Group. Allergy 2012;67: 147–57.
15. Craig T, Pursun EA, Bork K, et al. WAO guideline for the management of hereditary angioedema. World Allergy Organ J 2012;5:182–99.
16. Lang DM, Aberer W, Bernstein JA, et al. International consensus on hereditary and acquired angioedema. Ann Allergy Asthma Immunol 2012;109(6):395–402.
17. Craig TJ. Recent advances in hereditary angioedema self-administration treatment: summary of an international hereditary angioedema expert meeting. Int Arch Allergy Immunol 2013;161(Suppl 1):26–7.
18. Aygören-Pürsün E, Martinez-Saguer I, Rusicke E, et al. On demand treatment and home therapy of hereditary angioedema in Germany—the Frankfurt experience. Allergy Asthma Clin Immunol 2010;6(1):21.
19. Zingale LC, Beltrami L, Zanichelli A, et al. Angioedema without urticaria: a large clinical survey. CMAJ 2006;175(9):1065–70.
20. Bork K, Meng G, Staubach P, et al. Hereditary angioedema: new findings concerning symptoms, affected organs, and course. Am J Med 2006;119(3): 267–74.
21. Reshef A, Prematta MJ, Craig TJ. Signs and symptoms preceding acute attacks of hereditary angioedema: results of three recent surveys. Allergy Asthma Proc 2013;34(3):261–6.
22. Agostoni A, Aygören-Pürsün E, Binkley KE, et al. Hereditary and acquired angioedema: problems and progress: proceedings of the third C1 esterase inhibitor deficiency workshop and beyond. J Allergy Clin Immunol 2004;114(Suppl 3): S51–131.
23. Bygum A, Aygören-Pürsün E, Caballero T, et al. The hereditary angioedema burden of illness study in Europe (HAE-BOIS-Europe): background and methodology. BMC Dermatol 2012;12:4.
24. Lumry WR, Castaldo AJ, Vernon MK, et al. The humanistic burden of hereditary angioedema: impact on health-related quality of life, productivity, and depression. Allergy Asthma Proc 2010;31(5):407–14.
25. Cicardi M, Banerji A, Bracho F, et al. Icatibant, a new bradykinin-receptor antagonist, in hereditary angioedema. N Engl J Med 2010;363:532–41.
26. Cicardi M, Levy RJ, McNeil DL, et al. Ecallantide for the treatment of acute attacks in hereditary angioedema. N Engl J Med 2010;363:523–31.

27. Zuraw BL, Busse PJ, White M, et al. Nanofiltered C1 inhibitor concentrate for treatment of hereditary angioedema. N Engl J Med 2010;363:513–22.
28. Craig TJ, Levy RJ, Wasserman RL, et al. Efficacy of human C1 esterase inhibitor concentrate compared with placebo in acute hereditary angioedema attacks. J Allergy Clin Immunol 2009;124:801–8.
29. Zuraw B, Cicardi M, Levy RJ, et al. Recombinant human C1-inhibitor for the treatment of acute angioedema attacks in patients with hereditary angioedema. J Allergy Clin Immunol 2010;126(4):821–7.
30. Tourangeau LM, Castaldo AJ, Davis DK, et al. Safety and efficacy of physician-supervised self-managed C1 inhibitor replacement therapy. Int Arch Allergy Immunol 2012;157:417–24.
31. Levi M, Choi G, Picavet C, et al. Self-administration of C1-inhibitor concentrate in patients with hereditary or acquired angioedema caused by C1-inhibitor deficiency. J Allergy Clin Immunol 2006;117:904–8.
32. Longhurst HJ, Farkas H, Craig T, et al. HAE international home therapy consensus document. Allergy Asthma Clin Immunol 2010;6:22.
33. Riedl MA, Hurewitz DS, Levy R, et al. Nanofiltered C1 esterase inhibitor (human) for the treatment of acute attacks of hereditary angioedema: an open-label trial. Ann Allergy Asthma Immunol 2012;108(1):49–53.
34. Banta E, Horn P, Craig TJ. Response to ecallantide treatment of acute attacks of hereditary angioedema based on time to intervention: results from the EDEMA clinical trials. Allergy Asthma Proc 2011;32(4):319–24.
35. Maurer M, Aberer W, Bouillet L, et al, I O S Investigators. Hereditary angioedema attacks resolve faster and are shorter after early icatibant treatment. PLoS One 2013;8(2):e53773. http://dx.doi.org/10.1371/journal.pone.0053773.
36. Li HH, Campion M, Craig TJ, et al. Analysis of hereditary angioedema attacks requiring a second dose of ecallantide. Ann Allergy Asthma Immunol 2013;110(3):168–72.
37. Gower RG, Busse PJ, Aygören-Pürsün E, et al. Hereditary angioedema caused by C1-esterase inhibitor deficiency: a literature-based analysis and clinical commentary on prophylaxis treatment strategies. World Allergy Organ J 2011;4(Suppl 2):S9–21.
38. Gower RG, Lumry WR, Davis-Lorton MA, et al. Current options for prophylactic treatment of hereditary angioedema in the United States: patient-based considerations. Allergy Asthma Proc 2012;33(3):235–40.
39. Craig T, Riedl M, Dykewicz MS, et al. When is prophylaxis for hereditary angioedema necessary? Ann Allergy Asthma Immunol 2009;102:366–72.
40. Zuraw BL, Kalfus I. Safety and efficacy of prophylactic nanofiltered C1-inhibitor in hereditary angioedema. Am J Med 2012;125(9):938.e1–7.
41. Füst G, Farkas H, Csuka D, et al. Long-term efficacy of danazol treatment in hereditary angioedema. Eur J Clin Invest 2011;41(3):256–62.
42. Maurer M, Magerl M. Long-term prophylaxis of hereditary angioedema with androgen derivates: a critical appraisal and potential alternatives. J Dtsch Dermatol Ges 2011;9(2):99–107.
43. Gandhi PK, Gentry WM, Bottorff MB. Thrombotic events associated with C1 esterase inhibitor products in patients with hereditary angioedema: investigation from the United States Food and Drug Administration adverse event reporting system database. Pharmacotherapy 2012;32(10):902–9.
44. Bork K, Bygum A, Hardt J. Benefits and risks of danazol in hereditary angioedema: a long-term survey of 118 patients. Ann Allergy Asthma Immunol 2008;100(2):153–61.

45. Zilberberg MD, Nathanson BH, Jacobsen T, et al. Descriptive epidemiology of hereditary angioedema emergency department visits in the United States, 2006-2007. Allergy Asthma Proc 2011;32(5):390–4.
46. Frank MM. Hereditary angioedema: short-term prophylaxis for surgery. Allergy Asthma Proc 2012;33(4):303–4.

On-demand Therapy for Hereditary Angioedema

Jonathan A. Bernstein, MD

KEYWORDS

- Hereditary angioedema • On-demand therapies • Berinert • Ecallantide • Icatibant
- Ruconest • Guidelines

KEY POINTS

- Consensus guidelines recommend that all patients with HAE have acute on-demand therapy available.
- Three novel therapeutic agents for on-demand treatment are currently approved in the United States and 1 is pending approval.
- Self-administration or administration under supervision by a health care provider in the home setting is the preferred treatment approach because it allows the patient with HAE to treat attacks early after the onset of the angioedema attack.
- Future studies are needed to show that the widespread use of acute on-demand therapies improves quality of life and reduces the morbidity and mortality of patients with HAE.

INTRODUCTION

According to all consensus guidelines, patients with hereditary angioedema (HAE) caused by C1-INH deficiency should have access to on-demand treatment of acute HAE attacks.[1-3] A recent patientcentric guideline recommended that at least 2 on-demand therapies be available because patients often have heterogeneous responses to different medications (Zuraw B. correspondence; manuscript in press). Before 2009, in the United States, other than fresh frozen plasma, which has the inherent risk of viral transmission, there were no on-demand therapies available to treat acute HAE attacks.[4] Patients were managed symptomatically with hydration and pain medication; however, many patients just waited until their attacks resolved over several days. Over the past 5 years, 3 novel therapies approved by the US Food and Drug Administration (FDA) have become available with the indication for treating acute attacks of HAE, and 1 is currently pending approval (**Table 1**). This article provides an

Allergy Section, Division of Immunology, Department of Internal Medicine, College of Medicine, University of Cincinnati, 3255 Eden Avenue, Suite 350 ML#563, Cincinnati, OH 45267-0563, USA
E-mail address: Jonathan.Bernstein@uc.edu

Immunol Allergy Clin N Am 33 (2013) 487–494
http://dx.doi.org/10.1016/j.iac.2013.07.004
0889-8561/13/$ – see front matter © 2013 Elsevier Inc. All rights reserved.

Table 1
Acute on-demand novel therapies for HAE

Drug Name (Generic, Trade)	FDA Indications	Dosage	Mechanism	Anticipated Potential Side Effects
Plasma-derived nanofiltered C1-INH (Berinert-P, CSL Behring)	Acute attacks	20 U per kg intravenous	Inhibits plasma kallikrein, coagulation factors XIIa and XIa, C1s, C1r, MASP-1, MASP-2, and plasmin	Rare: risk of anaphylaxis Theoretic: transmission of infectious agent
Ecallantide (Kalbitor, Dyax)	Acute attacks	30 mg subcutaneous (administered as 3 injections of 10 mg/mL each)	Inhibits plasma kallikrein	Common: injection-site reactions Uncommon: antidrug antibodies, risk of anaphylaxis 2.7%
Icatibant (Firazyr, Shire)	Acute attacks	30 mg subcutaneous	Bradykinin B2 receptor antagonist	Common: discomfort at injection site
Recombinant human C1-INH (Rhucin, Pharming)	Acute attacks (pending FDA approval; approved by the EMA)	50–100 U per kg Intravenous	Inhibits plasma kallikrein, coagulation factors XIIa and XIa, C1s, C1r, MASP-1, MASP-2, and plasmin	Uncommon: risk of anaphylaxis in rabbit sensitized individuals rare

Abbreviation: EMA, European Medicines Agency.
Data from Zuraw BL. Clinical practice. Hereditary angioedema. N Engl J Med 2008;359(10):1027–36; and Zuraw BL, Bernstein JA, Lang DM, et al. A focused parameter update: hereditary angioedema, acquired C1 inhibitor deficiency, and angiotensin-converting enzyme inhibitor-associated angioedema. J Allergy Clin Immunol 2013;131(6):1491–3.e25.

overview of these therapies to enhance understanding of their mechanism of action and usefulness in the management of patients with HAE.

CONTACT PATHWAY AND SITES OF ACTION FOR ON-DEMAND TREATMENTS

Understanding the pathogenesis of HAE is essential for recognizing how acute on-demand therapies work.[4] **Fig. 1** shows the contact pathway and the points at which these novel therapies regulate C1-INH and kallikrein. Plasma-derived C1-INH works at several sites in the contact, complement, and plasmin pathways, but its two most important regulatory points are inhibiting the conversion of prekallikrein to kallikrein and inhibition of kallikrein's ability to convert high-molecular-weight kininogen to bradykinin, the putative mediator involved in causing the physiologic changes responsible for angioedema. Ecallantide, a recombinant kallikrein inhibitor, and icatibant, a bradykinin-2 receptor inhibitor, work by directly blocking kallikrein or inhibiting bradykinin 2 receptors, respectively.[4]

ON-DEMAND THERAPIES
Plasma-derived C1 Esterase Inhibitor (Berinert)

Berinert is a plasma-derived, nanofiltered, lyophilized, pasteurized C1-INH concentrate C1-INH (plasma-derived C1 esterase inhibitor [pdC1-INH]; CSL Behring, King of Prussia, PA), approved by the FDA in 2009 for the treatment of abdominal or facial HAE attacks, and more recently this indication was increased to include laryngeal attacks.[5,6] Berinert is also approved for self-administration by appropriately trained patients. Berinert has been available in Europe and Canada for more than 2 decades. Berinert is dosed at 20 U/kg intravenously.[5,6] Several clinical studies have shown the usefulness of pdC1-INH concentrate in the rapid and sustained treatment of HAE attacks. A large placebo-controlled trial (IMPACT 1 [International Multicenter Prospective Angioedema C1-Inhibitor Trial 1]) showed that onset of relief for facial or abdominal attacks occurred in a median of 0.5 hours, compared with 1.5 hours for placebo ($P = .003$). The time to onset of relief for severe attacks was 0.5 versus 13.5 hours.[5] The median time to complete resolution of all HAE symptoms, including pain, was 4.9 versus 7.8 hours ($P = .02$).[5] An open-label extension of this study

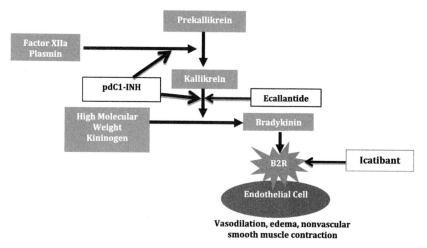

Fig. 1. Contact pathway and sites of activity for novel on-demand therapies.

(IMPACT 2) reported the results of patient assessments of 1085 attacks in all body locations.[7] The median time to onset of relief was 26.4 minutes for laryngeal attacks, 23.9 minutes for abdominal attacks, 28.8 minutes for facial attacks, and 25.8 minutes for peripheral attacks. The time to complete resolution of HAE symptoms was 5.8 hours for laryngeal attacks, 12.8 hours for abdominal attacks, 22.7 hours for peripheral attacks, and 26.6 hours for facial attacks. No rebound edema was observed.[7] Another study that compared the outcomes in 4834 severe abdominal attacks treated with pdC1-INH versus 17,444 untreated attacks found that the mean attack duration decreased from 92 to 40 hours with pdC1-INH treatment.[8] There were concomitant decreases in the associated events of nausea/vomiting (83.3%/41.8% vs 6.0%/11.0%) and cardiovascular collapse (3.5% vs 0.1%).[8] C1-esterase inhibitor was shown to be generally well tolerated. A recent study using patient data from the IMPACT 2 study investigated weight-based dosing in patients with HAE with body mass indexes of 18.4 to less than 25 kg/m^2 (normal weight), 25 to less than 30 kg/m^2 (overweight), and 30 to less than 40 kg/m^2 (obese). The median time to complete resolution of HAE attacks was 15.2 hours (95% confidence interval [CI], 9.3; 23.2) in normal-weight patients, 22.6 hours (95% CI, 11.3; 44.6) in overweight patients, and 11.0 hours (95% CI, 5.6; 23.6) in obese patients. There were no relevant differences in the incidence of AEs in patients with normal body weight (54%), overweight patients (30%), and obese patients (54%). These data support weight-based dosing in patients with HAE (abstract presented at the 2013 AAAAI meeting).

During early trials, dysgeusia was reported most often and more frequently than placebo (4.7% vs 2.4%) but otherwise Berinert was well tolerated with no evidence of thromboembolic disease.[9] Postmarketing data from around the world since 1985 have also reported few adverse events, including no transmission of infectious agents.[9]

Ecallantide (Kalbitor)

Ecallantide (Dyax Corp, Cambridge, MA) was also approved in the United States in 2009 for treatment of acute HAE peripheral, abdominal, and laryngeal attacks in patients 16 years of age and older.[10] Ecallantide is a recombinant protein generated by phage display technology that inhibits plasma kallikrein, a serine protease (see **Fig. 1**).[10] It is administered subcutaneously at a recommended dose of 30 mg, given as three 1-mL injections at least 2.5 cm from each other and away from the anatomic location of swelling. The dose can be repeated within 24 hours for persistent symptoms.[10]

Ecallantide has been evaluated for the acute treatment of moderate to severe HAE attacks in 2 large phase 3 placebo-controlled studies, EDEMA3 and EDEMA4.[11,12] The primary end point in each study was the change from baseline in mean symptom complex severity score, a point-in-time patient measure of symptom severity. Integrated analysis of data from both studies showed a significant improvement in median symptom complex severity score at all anatomic locations at 4 hours after dosing compared with placebo.[11,12] A post hoc analysis of the results of EDEMA4 concluded that, at 1 hour and 2 hours after dosing, subjects receiving ecallantide had a clinically meaningful trend toward greater improvement compared with the placebo group (P = not significant).[13]

Ecallantide seems to be well tolerated, with the most commonly reported adverse events being headache, nausea, diarrhea, pyrexia, injection-site reaction, and nasopharyngitis. In the EDEMA1, EDEMA3, and EDEMA4 studies with 255 patients, 10 patients had symptoms and clinical courses suggestive of anaphylaxis syndrome. Four subjects had a history of allergy/atopy, and 3 of the 4 tested positive for antiecallantide antibodies. All patients recovered without sequelae.[12,13] As a result of the risk of anaphylaxis with ecallantide, the product labeling contains a black-box warning indicating that it can only be administered by a trained health care professional equipped to manage anaphylaxis.[10] Postmarketing studies have not found an increase in the incidence of anaphylaxis with this medication. However, immunosurveillance studies have found that some patients produce specific immunoglobulin (Ig) G, IgA, or IgE to ecallantide, and these antibodies do not seem to functionally impair the activity of the medication or to correlate or predict an anaphylactic event should one occur.[10]

Icatibant (Firazyr)

Icatibant, a bradykinin-2 receptor antagonist, was approved by the FDA in August 2011 for the treatment of acute attacks of HAE in adults 18 years of age and older. Two phase 3 studies with subcutaneous icatibant were initially conducted. The For Angioedema Subcutaneous Treatment-1 (FAST-1) study compared icatibant with placebo in 56 subjects, and the FAST-2 study involved 74 patients and included an active comparator, tranexamic acid.[14] In FAST-2, median time to onset of symptom relief was significantly shorter with icatibant compared with tranexamic acid (2.0 vs 12.0 hours; $P<.001$), which supported regulatory approval by the FDA.[14] However, the FAST-1 study failed to show a significantly greater benefit relative to placebo. A post hoc analysis showed that early use of rescue medication in the FAST-1 placebo group may have been partially responsible for this finding, which necessitated an additional FAST-3 phase III, placebo-controlled study.[15] The results from FAST-3 were that icatibant was effective and well tolerated in acute HAE attacks. In patients with moderate to very severe cutaneous or abdominal symptoms, a 50% or greater reduction in symptom severity occurred within a median of 2.0 hours with icatibant compared with 19.8 hours for placebo ($P = .001$).[15] For laryngeal attacks, median time to 50% or more reduction in symptom severity was 2.5 hours with icatibant and 3.2 hours with placebo.[15] Overall, no subjects treated with icatibant required rescue medication, whereas 36% (16/45) of subjects using placebo did. Adverse event incidence was similar for icatibant and placebo (41% and 52%, respectively).[15] Icatibant is approved for self-administration as a single dose (30 mg subcutaneously) in the abdomen and can be stored at room temperature.

Recombinant Human C1-INH (Ruconest)

Ruconest, a highly purified human plasma protease C1 inhibitor is a recombinant protein expressed in the mammary gland of transgenic rabbits that is currently approved by the European Medicines Agency for treatment of acute HAE attacks and under review by the FDA.[16] Ruconest is structurally similar to the C1-INH gene but weighs less (67,000 kDa) because of lower glycosylation.[16] It is also functionally similar to human C1-INH because it can inhibit C1, plasma kallikrein, factor Xia, and factor XIIa.[16]

In 2 open-label, clinical studies on 9 patients with HAE treated with Ruconest for 13 angioedema attacks, the median time to onset of symptom relief was less than 60 minutes, whereas median time to minimal symptoms was less than 8 hours.[17] Visual analog scores for symptoms of peripheral attacks were obtained from 65 patients in all clinical trials. Treatment with Ruconest significantly decreased the duration of swelling, pain, and associated dysfunction of peripheral angioedema attacks in patients with HAE. Two separate randomized, double-blind, placebo-controlled clinical trials showed that median time to the beginning of symptom relief and median time to minimal symptoms was significantly improved with Ruconest.[18] Patients received Ruconest 100 U/kg, Ruconest 50 U/kg, or placebo. For the 100 U/kg, 50 U/kg, and placebo doses, patients reported onset of symptom relief at a median of 68 minutes, 122 minutes, and 258 minutes, respectively, and the time to minimal clinical symptoms of 245, 247, and 1098 minutes respectively were statistically significant relative to placebo ($P<.01$).[18]

The percentages of HAE attacks responding to 50 U/kg and 100 U/kg doses of Ruconest within 4 hours were 92% and 93%, respectively, compared with 41% with placebo.[18] Because no significant difference between 50 U/kg and 100 U/kg doses was observed, the 50 U/kg dose has been recommended for treatment of acute HAE attacks.

No drug-related adverse events or clinically relevant vital sign changes, electrocardiogram findings, or laboratory abnormalities (including hematological, biochemical, coagulation, viral serology, anti-C1-INH, and antibodies against rabbit milk protein) have been reported in clinical trials.[18,19] The most common side effect is headache. Transmission of rabbit or human viruses has not been observed.[20] There have been no detectable neutralizing antibodies.[16,18-20] One-hundred and thirty-seven healthy volunteers and patients with HAE were tested for the presence of IgE antibodies against 4 rabbit allergens and 10 other animal allergens after their last exposure to Ruconest.[16] Twenty-four of 137 (17.5%) subjects had at least one positive IgE antibody test result at baseline. Five subjects had a positive test against rabbit allergens. Three of the five subjects positive for IgE against rabbit allergens reported allergic symptoms after Ruconest exposure.[16] One healthy volunteer, who did not disclose a history of rabbit allergy and with the highest rabbit dander–specific IgE level (39 kU/L), had an anaphylactic reaction after the first exposure to Ruconest, which is the only allergic reaction reported thus far.[16] It is recommended to screen patients for antirabbit IgE before using Ruconest.[16]

Ruconest is freeze dried, preservative free, and contains 2100 units per vial after reconstitution in 14 mL of diluent.[16] One unit correlates with the amount of C1-INH in 1 mL of normal fresh plasma. Population pharmacokinetic modeling for Ruconest supports dosing of 50 U/kg up to 84 kg with a fixed dose of 4200 U for patients weighing more than 84 kg.[21] It is recommended that no more than 2 intravenous injections be administered within a 24-hour time span.[16]

SUMMARY

Hereditary angioedema is a chronic disorder that varies in severity over time for individual patients and between family members. Attack severity, frequency, and location all affect the management, assessment, and treatment of these patients. Regardless of whether or not patients are initiated on oral or intravenous prophylactic therapy, all patients with HAE are at increased risk for breakthrough attacks. For this reason, on-demand treatment of acute HAE attacks is a consensus recommendation by HAE experts.[2,3] The intent is to prevent life-threatening laryngeal attacks and/or debilitating abdominal or peripheral attacks, which invariably improve the quality of life of these patients by minimizing the impact of this disease on work and leisure activities.

Studies have uniformly shown that early administration of on-demand therapies after the beginning of swelling results in the best clinical outcomes and the least morbidity and mortality. Therefore, recent initiatives have focused on ensuring that these novel on-demand therapies can be self-administered or administered under the care of a trained health care professional at home. Recent surveys suggest that patients globally are favorable to this approach.[22] In addition, studies are currently investigating novel on-demand therapies that can be administered through preferable delivery routes (ie, subcutaneous or oral) and that will likely further improve management and control of HAE.

REFERENCES

1. Bowen T, Cicardi M, Bork K, et al. Hereditary angiodema: a current state-of-the-art review, VII: Canadian Hungarian 2007 international consensus algorithm for

the diagnosis, therapy, and management of hereditary angioedema. Ann Allergy Asthma Immunol 2008;100(1 Suppl 2):S30–40.

2. Cicardi M, Bork K, Caballero T, et al. Evidence-based recommendations for the therapeutic management of angioedema owing to hereditary C1 inhibitor deficiency: consensus report of an International Working Group. Allergy 2012;67: 147–57.

3. Zuraw BL, Bernstein JA, Lang DM, et al. A focused parameter update: hereditary angioedema, acquired C1 inhibitor deficiency, and angiotensin-converting enzyme inhibitor-associated angioedema. J Allergy Clin Immunol 2013;131(6): 1491–3.e25.

4. Zuraw BL. Clinical practice. Hereditary angioedema. N Engl J Med 2008;359(10): 1027–36.

5. Craig TJ, Lery RJ, Wasserman RL, et al. Efficacy of human C1 esterase inhibitor concentrate compared with placebo in acute hereditary angioedema attacks. J Allergy Clin Immunol 2009;124(4):801–8.

6. Epstein TG, Bernstein JA. Current and emerging management options for hereditary angioedema in the US. Drugs 2008;68(18):2561–73.

7. Craig TJ, Bewtra AK, Bahna SL, et al. C1 esterase inhibitor concentrate in 1085 hereditary angioedema attacks–final results of the I.M.P.A.C.T.2 study. Allergy 2011;66(12):1604–11.

8. Bork K, Meng G, Staubach P, et al. Treatment with C1 inhibitor concentrate in abdominal pain attacks of patients with hereditary angioedema. Transfusion 2005;45(11):1774–84.

9. Bork K, Barnstedt SE. Treatment of 193 episodes of laryngeal edema with C1 inhibitor concentrate in patients with hereditary angioedema. Arch Intern Med 2001;161(5):714–8.

10. Bernstein JA, Qazi M. Ecallantide: its pharmacology, pharmacokinetics, clinical efficacy and tolerability. Expert Rev Clin Immunol 2010;6(1):29–39.

11. Cicardi M, Lery RJ, McNeil DL, et al. Ecallantide for the treatment of acute attacks in hereditary angioedema. N Engl J Med 2010;363(6):523–31.

12. Levy RJ, Lumry WR, McNeil DL, et al. EDEMA4: a phase 3, double-blind study of subcutaneous ecallantide treatment for acute attacks of hereditary angioedema. Ann Allergy Asthma Immunol 2010;104(6):523–9.

13. Lunn M, Banta E. Ecallantide for the treatment of hereditary angiodema in adults. Clin Med Insights Cardiol 2011;5:49–54.

14. Cicardi M, Banerji A, Bracho F, et al. Icatibant, a new bradykinin-receptor antagonist, in hereditary angioedema. N Engl J Med 2010;363(6):532–41.

15. Lumry WR, Li HH, Levy RJ, et al. Randomized placebo-controlled trial of the bradykinin B(2) receptor antagonist icatibant for the treatment of acute attacks of hereditary angioedema: the FAST-3 trial. Ann Allergy Asthma Immunol 2011; 107(6):529–37.

16. Davis B, Bernstein JA. Conestat alfa for the treatment of angioedema attacks. Ther Clin Risk Manag 2011;7:265–73.

17. Plosker GL. Recombinant human c1 inhibitor (conestat alfa): in the treatment of angioedema attacks in hereditary angioedema. BioDrugs 2012;26(5):315–23.

18. Zuraw B, Cicardi M, Lery RJ, et al. Recombinant human C1-inhibitor for the treatment of acute angioedema attacks in patients with hereditary angioedema. J Allergy Clin Immunol 2010;126(4):821–7.e14.

19. Riedl MA, Lery RJ, Svez D, et al. Efficacy and safety of recombinant C1 inhibitor for the treatment of hereditary angioedema attacks: a North American open-label study. Ann Allergy Asthma Immunol 2013;110(4):295–9.

20. Hack CE, Relan A, Baboeram A, et al. Immunosafety of recombinant human C1-inhibitor in hereditary angioedema: evaluation of IgE antibodies. Clin Drug Investig 2013;33(4):275–81.
21. Farrell C, Haye SS, Relan A, et al. Population pharmacokinetics of recombinant human C1-inhibitor in patients with hereditary angioedema. Br J Clin Pharmacol 2013. [Epub ahead of print].
22. Caballero T, Sala-Cunill A, Cancian M, et al. Current status of implementation of self-administration training in various regions of Europe, Canada and the USA in the management of hereditary angioedema. Int Arch Allergy Immunol 2013; 161(Suppl 1):10–6.

Update on Preventive Therapy (Prophylaxis) for Hereditary Angioedema

Michael M. Frank, MD

KEYWORDS

- Hereditary angioedema • Prophylaxis • C1 inhibitor • Androgens • Antifibrinolytics

KEY POINTS

- The introduction of new and effective therapy to terminate acute attacks of angioedema in patients with hereditary angioedema has revolutionized the treatment landscape.
- Both attenuated androgens and inhibitors of fibrinolysis were found to provide effective preventive oral therapy in double blind studies, but each group causes unacceptable side effects or is inappropriate as therapy in some patients.
- In 2009, plasma derived C1 inhibitor was approved for prophylaxis in appropriate patients. The major disadvantage of this agent is that currently it must be administered by intravenous injection 2–3 times a week.
- Some patients require short term prophylaxis following trauma or prior to surgery. The drugs above have been used effectively in this setting and fresh frozen plasma has also proved to be useful prior to surgery.

INTRODUCTION

The introduction of new and effective therapy to terminate acute attacks of angioedema in patients with hereditary angioedema (HEA) has revolutionized the treatment landscape. In the past in America, prophylactic treatment to prevent the occurrence of attacks was the only reliable therapeutic option. Now there are multiple treatment modalities that have been proved to terminate attacks within hours and that have received Food and Drug Administration (FDA) approval. Nevertheless, there continues to be a need for long-term and short-term prophylaxis. Long-term prophylaxis is the designation given to long-term preventive therapy. Unlike the situation where each acute attack is treated, with effective prophylaxis attacks do not occur. Given the enormous morbidity of this disease, the high costs of the disease in terms of physician and hospital costs, and the costs of missed work and patient's being unable to work, prophylaxis to prevent attacks has always had high priority.[1] Short-term prophylaxis also

Department of Pediatrics, Duke University Medical Center, Erwin Road, Durham, NC 27710, USA
E-mail address: frank007@mc.duke.edu

Immunol Allergy Clin N Am 33 (2013) 495–503
http://dx.doi.org/10.1016/j.iac.2013.07.005
0889-8561/13/$ – see front matter © 2013 Elsevier Inc. All rights reserved.

immunology.theclinics.com

has a place in therapy when patients are not having attacks, but are in danger of having an attack in the near future. Thus, a patient undergoing surgery, having extensive dental work, or in a traumatic accident might be treated to prevent a possible future attack. The need for such treatment is clear. Many patients have attacks precipitated by trauma. If the trauma of dental manipulation or gum injection leads to angioedema starting in the mouth, airway compromise may result. In the days before prophylaxis, these patients learned to dread going to the dentist. Short-term prophylaxis addresses this possibility. Although as discussed, acute and effective therapy is now available if such swelling was to occur, the advantages of a preventative approach are obvious.

DEVELOPMENT OF THE OLDER AGENTS

Long-term preventive therapy for HAE was addressed long before we had knowledge of disease pathogenesis. A Swedish group, interested in defining diseases in which a newly described drug epsilon-aminocaproic acid (EACA), a fibrinolysis inhibitor, might be useful, administered the drug to patients with a wide variety of diseases.[2] They reported their experience in treating many diseases over a 5-year period. It was noted that a single patient with HAE seemed to improve on EACA. The report was noted by another Swedish group who treated a second patient with EACA and confirmed the finding.[3] This latter group was interested in the effect of EACA therapy on complement activation and histamine generation, the mediators thought at that time to be responsible for the angioedema. The group found no clear effect on either mediator pathway. They were unable to identify the mechanism by which EACA controlled the development of angioedema. A year later, Champion and Lachmann reported another family successfully treated with EACA.[4] Frank and colleagues[5] in 1972 conducted a double-blind study of the EACA prophylaxis, proving that EACA was far more effective than placebo in controlling attacks. In Europe, a cyclical derivative of EACA, tranexamic acid, was developed and has become the standard fibrinolysis inhibitor used in the treatment of HAE, because it is more convenient to use and has a better toxicity profile.[6] Blohme and colleagues studied the usefulness of this agent in HAE treatment and published a double-blind study showing that it is quite effective in prophylaxis. Tranexamic acid was not available in capsule form in America until recently and has not been widely used in this country. EACA has been used in this country, particularly for treatment of children, and is associated with a wide variety of long-term toxicities. With long-term EACA therapy, thrombosis has not been a problem in this investigator's experience, although it certainly is a theoretical problem, particularly in older individuals, but muscle aches and pains with weakness and markedly elevated creatine phosphokinase enzymes and a feeling of severe fatigue to the point of disability are commonly noted. It is now thought that EACA functions in HAE prophylaxis by inhibiting plasmin activation of kallikrein and that by interrupting the kinin generating cycle, it tends to inhibit attacks, but this has not been studied carefully and it remains a supposition. Because use of EACA use was clearly associated with great difficulty over time, more effective and safer prophylactic agents were needed.

Frank and colleagues[7] were struck by the endocrinologic aspects of HAE. The disease, inherited as an autosomal dominant trait, is equal in incidence in men and women and becomes worse at the time of puberty in both sexes. Nevertheless, they noted that it is made much more severe by estrogens, such as those in birth control tablets and most patients who come to a clinic are women. In their experience, most women were much improved clinically during the latter part of pregnancy and many of the patients who they were observing said that the last trimester of pregnancy was the best period that they had experienced clinically in many years. They never had attacks precipitated by the trauma of delivery, although some of the patients often had attacks precipitated by other trauma. These findings were not uniformly true and a minority of the women seen in Frank's clinic became much more severely ill during pregnancy. The observation is of interest because German investigators have reported that German women have no clear change in severity in pregnancy and the Australians have reported that their experience is similar to that in Frank's clinic.[8] A recent European report based on a questionnaire sent to a large number of European women came to the conclusion that about one-third of patients got better, one-third became worse, and about one-third had no change.[9] The reasons for these differences are unknown, but it is of interest that pregnant women in America were on no therapy, whereas women in Germany had available purified C1 inhibitor to rapidly terminate attacks.

Because progesterone rises progressively during pregnancy and falls precipitously on delivery, Frank's group first studied the effect of progesterone as prophylaxis in a small group of patients. The essentially negative study was never published. Although they noted that all of the treated women felt better and reported fewer symptoms, there was no decrease in the frequency of attacks when the drug was compared with placebo. Other more recent uncontrolled studies suggest that some women will respond well to this agent.

Our group set out to find a gonadotropin inhibitor that would decrease the synthesis of estrogens in men and women. The drug chosen for study was danazol, a gonadotropin inhibitor that was being developed as a contraceptive for women and that was felt to be safely used in women. In a double-blind study, it was shown that this drug is extremely effective in prophylaxis of HAE (**Table 1**) and in some patients, surprisingly, raised the blood level of C1 inhibitor to normal.[10] The drug was so effective that it was approved by FDA for HAE prophylaxis on the basis of study of these 9 patients. Because patients are heterozygotes, they have one normal gene allele and one abnormal gene; the finding suggests that the functional output of the normal allele increases on danazol therapy. There are data to support and refute this suggestion and the question is not settled. Over the next years, it was quickly discovered that all of the 17-methylated and attenuated androgens are useful in the prophylaxis of HAE. Testosterone itself is not effective. A similar androgen, stanozolol, also received FDA approval for HAE therapy following a double-blind study, but it is currently only obtained in the United States through compounding pharmacies.[11] Interestingly, it also has been found that androgens increase the level of bradykinin degrading enzymes like aminopeptidase P.[12] At present it seems that androgens both decrease the formation of bradykinin by increasing C1 inhibitor levels and increase its degradation by degrading enzymes, thereby preventing these bradykinin-initiated attacks, but this is by no means settled.

Table 1
Results of a double-blind study of the use of danazol versus placebo in HAE prophylaxis. Patients received drug or placebo for about a month. At the end of each study period, they went on to the next random drug or placebo course. If the patient experienced an attack, the course that they were on was deemed a failure and they continued immediately to the next random course. The marked effect of danazol in prophylaxis is evident

	Danazol Treatment Results		
	Total Courses	Attack-Free Courses	Attacks
Placebo	46	3	43
Danazol	42	41	1
Total	88	44	44

Although the original FDA approval of danazol was based on the results in very few patients, the drug has come to be used around the world and there is now a great deal of clinical experience with its use. In an interesting study in 2008, Bork and Barnstedt[13] reported a retrospective analysis of the Danish and German experience in treating 118 patients for an average of 11 years. The drug was effective in the vast majority of patients; 54 of 118 (45.8%) patients became symptom free or had 1 attack or less per year. In almost all of the other patients the disease became milder. The frequency of acute attacks was reduced to 16.2% of the pretreatment number. Adverse events (weight gain, virilization, menstrual irregularities, headache, depression, and/or liver abnormalities) were noted in 98 patients, but in general were mild and the drug was withdrawn in 30. Because the drug was developed as a contraceptive, many of these are not true side effects but relate to the expected physiologic action of the drug. Interestingly, most of the patients who discontinued the drug because of side effects did so in the first 2 years after treatment was started. A more recent study of the German and Hungarian experience makes other interesting points.[14] It is pointed out that some individuals with borderline hypertension may become hypertensive on danazol treatment. Marked differences were found between the German and Hungarian cohort. The German's had 3 times the number of abdominal attacks when compared with the Hungarians and the Hungarians had more laryngeal attacks. Danazol did not become less effective over time in the German cohort and did become somewhat less effective in the Hungarians. It is this investigators' unpublished experience that if danazol becomes less effective over time, treatment can be discontinued for several months and that the drug will be more effective again when it is restarted.

As mentioned earlier, there are many side effects associated with danazol therapy and most of these side effects are associated with the other attenuated androgens as well.[15] Almost all patients note weight gain and many patients have lipid abnormalities.[16,17] Plasma low-density lipoprotein and cholesterol have been noted to be increased and high-density lipoprotein (HDL) levels to fall. One study suggests that the incidence of atherosclerosis rises, but the study only presents data on lipid levels, which are in keeping with such a suggestion.[17] Because the patients are on these agents for prolonged periods, these are not minor complications. In a more limited but much more complete study of lipids in 17 patients who were on danazol for an average of more than 2 years at an average dose of 170 mg/d compared with controls, the effects were less impressive.[18] It was pointed out that the values in this study were corrected for body mass index, a correction not applied in earlier studies. There were no changes in HDL-cholesterol or carotid intima-media thickness in this study. On the other hand, patients had signs of coagulation pathway activation.

Some patients develop liver function abnormalities with abnormal liver enzymes on androgen therapy. There is considerable variation from study to study. For example, in a long-term study of 70 Italian patients with HAE, no significant liver abnormalities were noted.[16] On the other hand, in a handful of patients liver cysts or carcinomas have been reported. Some patients develop myopathies, hematuria, headaches, abnormal menses, increased or decreased libido, hair loss or gain, or anxiety reactions. In general, all of these side effects are quite mild and it is unusual for patients to come off danazol therapy because of side effects.[19] Nevertheless, the side effect list is long and of concern. When patients are treated, the dose is progressively lowered until patients are having occasional attacks, because the severity of the side effects is dose-related.

The patient's clinical signs and symptoms must be followed carefully, but the levels of blood proteins like C1 inhibitor and C4 are not used to determine clinical effectiveness. It must be noted that impeded androgens are not effective in some patients.

They usually are not used in children because of the possibility of premature closure of the epiphyses but there are studies of danazol and oxandrolone use in childhood.[20,21] They are not used in pregnancy, particularly in the first trimester, because of the danger of masculinization of the fetus. They are ineffective in some people. In addition, there are no intramuscular or intravenous (IV) preparations. Testosterone itself is not effective. The drugs must be given orally, and if a patient is having an abdominal attack with edematous gastrointestinal mucosa, the drugs may not be absorbed. Although the androgens are useful in prophylaxis, they are not useful in acute therapy. They do not have maximal effect for about 48 hours.

For all of these reasons, it was important that other forms of therapy be developed that have fewer side effects and be useful in all patients. There was a long history of using plasma-purified C1 inhibitor to treat acute HAE attacks and attention turned back to this agent for both acute treatment and prophylaxis.

C1 INHIBITOR USE IN PROPHYLAXIS

Three independent groups began the process of purifying C1 inhibitor from pooled plasma of thousands of donors in the mid 1970s. All 3 groups had extensive experience in purifying gamma globulin from plasma and had available facilities for processing plasma in large quantities. The Dutch Red Cross in the Netherlands, Behring Pharmaceuticals in Germany, and the American Red Cross in the United States all successfully purified the protein. C1 inhibitor was reported effective in treating HAE attacks in studies of all 3 products. Gadek and colleagues[10] reported on the biochemical effect of the American Red Cross C1 inhibitor on C1 inhibitor and C4 blood levels in 8 patients with HAE in 1980 and showed that in 5 patients who were having attacks at the time of infusion, the agent terminated the attacks. Agostoni and Cicardi studied the Dutch Red Cross product and reported that it was effective in terminating an attack.[22] It is this product that in a modern version has been approved for prophylaxis in the United States. Similarly, Bork studied the CSL Behring product and showed that it was effective in anecdotal report.[23] All of the early studies relied on historical experience to determine effectiveness of the agents, and it was important that a double-blind study to compare C1 inhibitor to placebo be performed in this highly variable disease. Such a study was reported by Waytes and colleagues[24] in 1996. This study compared with placebo yet another C1 inhibitor product prepared by Immuno of Austria. They reported the effectiveness both in terminating attacks and, in an inpatient portion of the study, in prophylaxis of disease. In the prophylaxis part of the study, they showed in 6 patients with severe disease who had not responded to conventional treatment that this agent given at 25 units/kg every 3 days for a total of 5 infusions was highly effective in prophylaxis. They followed the blood level of C1 inhibitor and C4 over the entire period of treatment. Blood levels of C1 inhibitor rose to normal immediately following infusion and by 3 days after infusion were again markedly depressed, illustrating the short half life of this plasma protein. As in earlier studies, the blood levels of C4 came back to normal more slowly, but then remained normal for the duration of the study. Placebo infusions did not affect either C1 inhibitor of C4 levels. Patient's attacks decreased by 60% compared with placebo but interestingly they did not decrease to zero.

The CSL Behring product, Berinert, was first licensed in Germany in 1985 and has been approved or licensed in Europe since that time. The Dutch Red Cross serum protein purification laboratory was merged into Sanquin in 2003. In 1989 heat treatment was added and more recently nanofiltration was added to further ensure sterility. These 2 products have been available in Europe for acute treatment of HAE attacks for several decades and, although they were never studied in a double blind fashion, many reports attest to their effectiveness. They were never approved by the US FDA and they were never available in the United States. With the onset of the AIDS epidemic in 1980, the American Red Cross turned its attention away from HAE and their C1 inhibitor product was no longer made.

TRIALS OF THE CURRENTLY APPROVED C1 INHIBITOR PREPARATION

In 2008, nanofiltered, plasma-derived C1 inhibitor distributed by ViroPharma was approved for prophylaxis of patients with frequent or severe attacks. A relatively similar C1 inhibitor preparation prepared by CSL Behring was approved a year later for treatment of acute attacks. Other reviewers will discuss therapy for acute disease, but it should be remembered that C1 inhibitor is a physiologic protein that controls many mediator systems in blood. It is capable of down-regulating clotting factor XIIa and plasmin generation as well as kallikrein generation and complement activation. Under normal circumstances, the protein prevents untoward generation of bradykinin by down-regulating activation of the kinin generating system. The only currently available agent that has been studied in a controlled prophylaxis trial is the Dutch Red Cross agent, now imported by the pharmaceutical company ViroPharma and sold under the brand name Cinryze.[25] The prophylaxis portion of the trial followed a blinded trial of acute therapy. Patients had a preliminary screening visit to establish their diagnosis as types 1 or 2 HAE and then participated in an acute treatment trial. Following this portion of the study and, while the patients were still blinded with respect to the drugs they had received, they entered the prophylaxis trial. The placebo controlled trial that was conducted was a double-blind cross-over study in which patients received either C1 inhibitor at 1000 units or placebo intravenously every 3 to 4 days for a 12-week period and then crossed over for an additional 12 weeks to receive the alternate agent. If patients on any agent had an angioedema attack, they were eligible to receive in an unblinded fashion 1000 units of C1 inhibitor as rescue medication and they then resumed the study. The drug proved effective at decreasing attack frequency and duration as well as attack severity, and the number of open label rescue therapy treatments was markedly reduced in patients receiving drug compared with placebo (**Fig. 1**). Side effects were minimal. The study confirmed that psychological factors have a major effect on attack frequency in HAE. An interesting patient in the prophylaxis study actually had more attacks during treatment with Cinryze than on prophylaxis because of difficult events in her life. When her life became more normal, her attack frequency decreased markedly. It is interesting that HAE patients in all double-bind trials tend to have a higher attack frequency than those being treated with known effective agents. When the patient is perfectly confident that the agent will terminate attacks, their response rate is markedly higher. These factors must be kept in mind in considering treatment regimens in patients with HAE. In October of 2008, Cinryze was approved by the FDA at 1000 units IV bi-weekly for prophylaxis.

THEORETICAL PROBLEMS AND ADVANTAGES

All plasma products have a risk of infection. The risk is certainly minor with currently available C1 inhibitor products because they have been used in Europe for decades and no infection has been observed. Both start with the blood from healthy American donors and go through potent virus reduction purifications. At present, C1 inhibitor is administered IV, which is a disadvantage. Both CSL Behring and ViroPharma are examining the use of subcutaneous (SQ) injection of C1 inhibitor. As this product becomes available it should have the advantage of providing more stable blood levels of

Endpoints Results: Median of within Patient

Percent Differences (95% CI)

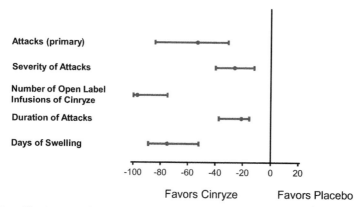

Fig. 1. The effectiveness of Cinryze prophylaxis in preventing HAE attacks. Shown is the statistical analysis of the activity of Cinryze in decreasing attack frequency, severity, duration, days of swelling, and open-label rescue treatments in the prophylaxis study. The effect is marked but as in other studies attack frequency did not decrease to zero.

protein and be more convenient to use. They may be more effective than the IV product which, because of its relatively short half life, does not maintain normal levels, even if administered every 3 to 4 days. Rate of absorption is a rate-limiting step in the use of SQ C1 inhibitor and the ViroPharma product is being studied with added hyaluronidase to improve absorption. Because patients are all heterozygotes and synthesize some normal C1 inhibitor, allergy to the administered product is unlikely. Because this is the normal physiologic protein, presumably it will provide normal physiologic regulation.

SHORT-TERM THERAPY

As mentioned earlier, there are circumstances where it is important to prevent attacks. It is both the patient experience and is reported that laryngeal attacks may follow tooth extraction.[13] Fresh frozen plasma (FFP) as a source of C1 inhibitor has been recommended for the treatment of acute attacks.[26] We do not recommend FFP for treatment of acute attacks although it is clear that the vast majority of patients do note termination of attacks. FFP supplies high-molecular-weight (HMW) kininogen and prekallikrein, 2 proteins that are consumed during kinin generation. The cleavage of administered HMW kininogen in some patients generates additional bradykinin. The supply of fresh substrate for kinin generation may make attacks worse before the attack starts to resolve and the authors have seen patients develop more severe angioedema following FFP. Nevertheless, when the patient is not having an angioedema attack, it is safe to give FFP, we and others have reported on its use in dental and other types of surgery.[27,28] Two units of FFP in our hands have prevented all acute angioedema attacks. Others have advocated 1 week of attenuated androgen therapy starting 1 week before these procedures. Androgens like danazol, even when used at high dose, usually have minimal side effects if only used for a week and these disappear rapidly. They have been used successfully before dental and surgical procedures.[29] Obviously, the new C1 inhibitor preparations also provide protection in these situations. In providing the deficient protein, while being free of kinin substrates, these agents are ideal for preventing attacks. In every case, products should be made available that reliable terminate unexpected acute attacks.

SUMMARY

In the period of one professional lifetime, the field has gone from an incomplete clinical picture of the syndrome to a complete clinical picture, to an understanding of the gene defect and the pathophysiology of the disease, and to having drugs available for acute therapy and for prophylaxis that bring this disease under control. The lot of patients with HAE is markedly improved.

REFERENCES

1. Wilson DA, Bork K, Shea EP, et al. Economic costs associated with acute attacks and long-term management of hereditary angioedema. Ann Allergy Asthma Immunol 2010;104(4):314–20.
2. Nilsson IM, Andersson L, Bjorkman SE. Epsilon-aminocaproic acid (E-ACA) as a therapeutic agent based on 5 year's clinical experience. Acta Med Scand Suppl 1966;448:1–46.
3. Lundh B, Laurell AB, Wetterqvist H, et al. A case of hereditary angioneurotic oedema, successfully treated with epsilon-aminocaproic acid. Studies on C'1 esterase inhibitor, C'1 activation, plasminogen level and histamine metabolism. Clin Exp Immunol 1968;3(7):733–45.
4. Champion RH, Lachmann PJ. Hereditary angio-oedema treated with E-amino-caproic acid. Br J Dermatol 1969;81(10):763–5.
5. Frank MM, Sergent JS, Kane MA, et al. Epsilon aminocaproic acid therapy of hereditary angioneurotic edema. A double-blind study. N Engl J Med 1972;286(15):808–12.
6. Blohme G. Treatment of hereditary angioneurotic oedema with tranexamic acid. A random double-blind cross-over study. Acta Med Scand 1972;192(4):293–8.
7. Frank MM, Gelfand JA, Atkinson JP. Hereditary angioedema: the clinical syndrome and its management. Ann Intern Med 1976;84(5):580–93.
8. Chinniah N, Katelaris CH. Hereditary angioedema and pregnancy. Aust N Z J Obstet Gynaecol 2009;49(1):2–5.
9. Bouillet L, Longhurst H, Boccon-Gibod I, et al. Disease expression in women with hereditary angioedema. Am J Obstet Gynecol 2008;199(5):484.e1–4.
10. Gadek JE, Hosea SW, Gelfand JA, et al. Replacement therapy in hereditary angioedema: successful treatment of acute episodes of angioedema with partly purified C1 inhibitor. N Engl J Med 1980;302(10):542–6.
11. Sheffer AL, Fearon DT, Austen KF. Clinical and biochemical effects of stanozolol therapy for hereditary angioedema. J Allergy Clin Immunol 1981;68(3):181–7.
12. Drouet C, Desormeaux A, Robillard J, et al. Metallopeptidase activities in hereditary angioedema: effect of androgen prophylaxis on plasma aminopeptidase P. J Allergy Clin Immunol 2008;121(2):429–33.
13. Bork K, Barnstedt SE. Laryngeal edema and death from asphyxiation after tooth extraction in four patients with hereditary angioedema. J Am Dent Assoc 2003;134(8):1088–94.
14. Farkas H, Czaller I, Csuka D, et al. Long-term efficacy of danazol treatment in hereditary angioedema. Eur J Clin Invest 2010;41(3):256–62.
15. Zurlo JJ, Frank MM. The long-term safety of danazol in women with hereditary angioedema. Fertil Steril 1990;54(1):64–72.

16. Cicardi M, Bergamaschini L, Cugno M, et al. Long-term treatment of hereditary angioedema with attenuated androgens: a survey of a 13-year experience. J Allergy Clin Immunol 1991;87(4):768–73.

17. Szeplaki G, Varga L, Valentin S, et al. Adverse effects of danazol prophylaxis on the lipid profiles of patients with hereditary angioedema. J Allergy Clin Immunol 2005;115(4):864–9.

18. Birjmohun RS, Kees Hovingh G, Stroes ES, et al. Effects of short-term and long-term danazol treatment on lipoproteins, coagulation, and progression of atherosclerosis: two clinical trials in healthy volunteers and patients with hereditary angioedema. Clin Ther 2008;30(12):2314–23.

19. Bork K, Bygum A, Hardt J. Benefits and risks of danazol in hereditary angioedema: a long-term survey of 118 patients. Ann Allergy Asthma Immunol 2008; 100(2):153–61.

20. Church JA. Oxandrolone treatment of childhood hereditary angioedema. Ann Allergy Asthma Immunol 2004;92(3):377–8.

21. Farkas H, Harmat G, Fust G, et al. Clinical management of hereditary angio-oedema in children. Pediatr Allergy Immunol 2002;13(3):153–61.

22. Agostoni A, Bergamaschini L, Martignoni G, et al. Treatment of acute attacks of hereditary angioedema with C1-inhibitor concentrate. Ann Allergy 1980;44(5): 299–301.

23. Bork K, Witzke G. Hereditares angioneurotisches Odem. Klinik sowie erweiterte diagnostische und therapeutische Moglichkeiten. Dtsch Med Wochenschr 1979;104(11):405–9 [in German].

24. Waytes AT, Rosen FS, Frank MM. Treatment of hereditary angioedema with a vapor-heated C1 inhibitor concentrate. N Engl J Med 1996;334:1630–4.

25. Zuraw BL, Busse PJ, White M, et al. Nanofiltered C1 inhibitor concentrate for treatment of hereditary angioedema. N Engl J Med 2010;363(6):513–22.

26. Pickering RJ, Good RA, Kelly JR, et al. Replacement therapy in hereditary angioedema. Successful treatment of two patients with fresh frozen plasma. Lancet 1969;1(7590):326–30.

27. Wall RT, Frank M, Hahn M. A review of 25 patients with hereditary angioedema requiring surgery. Anesthesiology 1989;71(2):309–11.

28. Jaffe CJ, Atkinson JP, Gelfand JA, et al. Hereditary angioedema: the use of fresh frozen plasma for prophylaxis in patients undergoing oral surgery. J Allergy Clin Immunol 1975;55(6):386–93.

29. Bowen T, Hebert J, Ritchie B, et al. Canadian 2003 International Consensus Algorithm for the diagnosis, therapy, and management of hereditary angioedema. J Allergy Clin Immunol 2004;114(3):629–37.

Hereditary Angioedema in Women
Specific Challenges

Laurence Bouillet, MD, PhD[a],*, Anne Gompel, MD, PhD[b,c]

KEYWORDS

- Hereditary angioedema • Female • Estrogen • Progestin

KEY POINTS

- Women with hereditary angioedema present with more frequent and more severe attacks.
- Exogenous and endogenous estrogens often worsen hereditary angioedema.
- Progestin is a promising long-term prophylactic treatment of women with hereditary angioedema.

Hereditary angioedema (HAE) is a rare disease that is transmitted by an autosomal dominant gene.[1] However, studies show a preponderance of female sufferers.[2,3] This predominance can be explained by women displaying severe symptoms more often than men and thus they are more often diagnosed.[3,4] During their lifetimes, symptoms can fluctuate, with periods when the disease worsens and periods when it gets better. In women, the age at which the first symptoms appear often correlates with the onset of puberty, and subsequent flare-up often corresponds with gynecologic events: contraception, pregnancies, and so forth. Pregnancy aggravates symptoms in 40% of cases, and exogenous estrogen often aggravates the disease.[5] Some women report that their symptoms coincide with their periods.[6] Estroprogestin contraception increases the frequency of attacks in 63% to 80% of women,[7,8] and hormone replacement treatment can trigger the appearance of the first symptoms.[9] In contrast, long-term treatment with a contraceptive progestin could reduce the frequency of attacks.[10] This is the evidence that has prompted this article, which discusses how women with HAE are treated.

The authors have no conflict of interest for this article.
[a] National Reference Centre for Angioedema (CREAK), Internal Medicine Department, Grenoble University Hospital, Joseph Fourier Grenoble 1 University, Cedex 09, Grenoble 38043, France; [b] Department of Gynecology Endocrinology, Port Royal Cochin Hospital (AP-HP), Paris Descartes University, 53 Avenue de l'observatoire, Paris, France; [c] National Reference Centre for Angioedema (CREAK)
* Corresponding author.
E-mail address: lbouillet@chu-grenoble.fr

PHYSIOPATHOLOGY

Visy and colleagues[11] showed that, in 44 women with HAE, the frequency of attacks correlated with estrogen and progesterone levels. The female sexual hormones act on several proteins, including the kallikrein-kinin system. In ovariectomized rats, B2 bradykinin receptor messenger RNA levels are reduced.[12] Estrogen substitution restores these levels and increases transcription of factor XII, kallikrein, and high-molecular-weight kininogen (HMWK).[13]

Levels of factor XII, prekallikrein, kallikrein, and HMWK are all increased in healthy women taking an estroprogestin pill.[14,15] This increase is associated with a proportional decrease in C1 inhibitor (C1Inh).

An increase in factor XII and kallikrein is also observed in healthy women taking oral estrogens.[16] In addition, the activity of the main kinase (angiotensin-converting enzyme) decreases, and bradykinin levels increase in these women.[17]

These data lead us to conclude that estrogens (both endogenous and exogenous) can disrupt the kallikrein-kinin pathway to favor the production of kininogenases (**Table 1**).

PHENOTYPES IN WOMEN

The HAE type that seems to be the most sensitive to female hormones is C1Inh-normal HAE (type III).[18,19] In 2000, the first cases of this form of the disease were described in women for whom attacks occurred only when taking the pill or during pregnancy.[20-22] Since then, the number of cases identified has increased, and symptomatic men have been identified. Three patient profiles have now been defined for type III AE[23,24]:

- Estrogen-dependent women: symptoms only occur when taking the pill and/or during pregnancies.
- Estrogen-sensitive women: symptoms are aggravated by taking the pill and/or during pregnancies. In addition, attacks continue to occur outside these specific contexts.
- Estrogen-insensitive women: the disease is not aggravated by exogenous estrogen and/or pregnancy.

Similar profiles are also described for C1Inh-deficit HAE (types I and II). Women with type I or II HAE are often sensitive to estrogens, with aggravation of their symptoms during pregnancy (40%) and/or when taking the pill (80%).[5,6]

PREGNANCY

The rate of spontaneous miscarriage in women with HAE is the same as for the general population. Thus, no specific fertility problems are associated with the disease.[5]

Table 1	
Influence of estrogens on the kallikrein-kinin pathway	
Increase	**Decrease**
Factor XII	C1Inh
Prekallikrein, kallikrein	ACE activity
HMWK, bradykinin	—
B2 receptor	—

Abbreviation: ACE, angiotensin converting enzyme.

In 40% of cases, pregnancy exacerbates HAE symptoms, with an increased frequency of attacks, particularly during the third trimester.[5,25,26] An increase in attacks can also occur as soon as the first days of pregnancy.

The delivery often goes smoothly, but some cases of stillborn children have been described for women with type normal C1Inh HAE.[27] Cesarean section is not systematically indicated. The rate of vaginal delivery is the same as for the general population.[5] Epidural and rachianesthesia present no particular problems or contraindications.[28]

When the patient has had a large number of attacks during her pregnancy, prophylactic measures should be taken by administering concentrated C1Inh before labor. If prophylactic measures are not taken, C1Inh should be available in the labor room in case it is needed.[28]

Danazol is commonly used to treat HAE, but its use is strictly contraindicated throughout pregnancy.[28] Other treatments, including icatibant, recombinant C1Inh, and ecallantide, are not recommended (because of lack of data).[28] However, tranexamic acid can be prescribed. No fetal abnormalities have been found in teratogenic studies in animals. This compound has been found (in the literature and our experience) to be safe for both mother and child.[29,30] Concentrated C1Inh should be used to treat severe attacks, or as a long-term prophylactic treatment if attacks are frequent, and this treatment has also been found to be safe for mother and child (in the literature and our experience).[25,26,29,31,32]

HAE does not require prenatal diagnosis. Diagnosis can be performed at birth using cord blood and a search for the familial mutation (if the parents' genotypes are known), or from 6 months of age using weighted functional C1Inh assays.

Lactation is allowed. Danazol, icatibant, recombinant C1Inh, and ecallantide should be avoided when breastfeeding, and only C1Inh concentrates have been shown to be safe.[28] Tranexamic acid can be prescribed given that less than 1% of the maternal dose is recovered in the milk.

IN VITRO FERTILIZATION

These procedures are usually associated with large and rapid increase in endogenous estrogen during ovarian stimulation. Ovarian stimulation by gonadotropins is usually combined with an antigonadotropic agent, which helps to increase the ovarian response to the gonadotropin stimulation. In patients with HAE, the pill should be avoided. In vitro fertilization should be performed as often as possible during spontaneous cycles, when estradiol is less likely to reach high levels and the risk of hyperstimulation is lower. If an ovarian stimulation is necessary, it could be performed using gonadotrophin-releasing hormone (GnRH) agonist or a progestin. Danazol is able at high dose to be antigonadotropic (600 mg/d) and could be used with reimplantation of the embryos in another cycle than one with ovocyte retrieval (Anne Gompel, MD, PhD, personal communication, 2012).

CONTRACEPTION

Estroprogestin contraceptives aggravate HAE symptoms in 63% to 80% of women with HAE.[5-7] Therefore, their use is not recommended for women with this disease. Copper intrauterine devices (IUDs) are well tolerated but remain neutral at the hormonal levels.[5]

Progestins are more than contraceptives; they are a long-term prophylaxis for women with HAE. Progestin-only contraceptives are a suitable alternative to the pill.[28] Progestins are well tolerated in these women, and they can improve symptoms by reducing the frequency of attacks.[10] This finding was especially true for potent anti-gonadotropic agents. By decreasing endogenous estradiol secretion they help to provide a more favorable hormonal context for these women.[10] We have shown that they could also be a prophylactic treatment of HAE, because 82% of women taking potent progestin report a decrease in the frequency of attacks. Thirty-six percent of women have no more attacks when taking this hormone.[10] In addition, for the antigonadotropic progestin, normethyltestosterone derivates are mild androgens and thus could in theory be associated, when administrated at high dose, with an even greater effect.[28] However, they have not so far been systematically evaluated. Low-dose progestin-only pills, as well as implants and levonorgestrel IUDs, are well tolerated in 60% of users but they can worsen attacks by inducing endogenous estrogen production in some patients.[10]

MENOPAUSE

The onset of the menopause improves symptoms for very few women (13%); a larger proportion (32%) experience aggravation.[9] One hypothesis explaining this outcome is that, although estrogen levels decrease at the menopause, ovarian androgens also decrease, and some women could be more sensitive to their protective effect.

BREAST CANCER

HAE is not associated with an increase in the incidence of breast cancer, which is the same as for the general population.[5] If breast cancer is diagnosed, hormone therapy should be carefully considered because tamoxifen has been linked to exacerbated symptoms.[33] In premenopausal women, tamoxifen is usually well tolerated as an anti-estrogen but, when combined with a GnRH agonist, it becomes an estrogen agonist and can promote attacks. After menopause, aromatase inhibitors are the first-line adjuvant hormone therapy and do not seem to exacerbate the disease.[33]

ATTENUATED ANDROGENS

Attenuated androgens (danazol, stanozolol, and so forth) are an effective treatment of C1Inh-deficit HAE.[34] However, their efficacy should be weighed against their metabolic and endocrine side effects, which can be severe.[35] These effects are particularly prevalent in women: virilization (6%), weight gain (30%), acne (7%), and menstrual irregularity (30%). Alopecia, hirsutism, and mammary hypotrophia have also been reported, but more sporadically.[35,36] The side effects are often dose dependent, and a balance may be achieved with small weekly doses.[37] In our practice, good tolerance and efficacy has been achieved with 200 mg danazol 3 times per week. Danazol is not a contraceptive and, even though it may cause amenorrhea, women can still get

Table 2	
Circumstances of worsening or improvement of HAE in women	
Worsening	**Improvement**
Estrogen-progestin contraceptives	Progestin
Menopause	Menopause
Pregnancy	Androgens
Hormone replacement therapy	—
Tamoxifen	—

pregnant when using it. In addition, danazol should not be used during pregnancy or breastfeeding.

SUMMARY

Knowledge of HAE has progressed considerably in recent years, and gender specificities have been identified. This progress has resulted in better therapeutic management of female patients (**Table 2**). The context of pregnancy is better understood and this reassures patients. Progress remains to be made in the area of long-term treatments. However, the potential of progestin has suggested new possibilities.

REFERENCES

1. Longhurst H, Cicardi M. Hereditary angio-oedema. Lancet 2012;379:474–81.
2. Agostoni A, Cicardi M. Hereditary and acquired C1 inhibitor deficiency: biological and clinical characteristics in 235 patients. Medicine 1992;71:206–15.
3. Bork K, Meng G, Staubach P, et al. Hereditary angioedema: new findings concerning symptoms, affected organs and course. Am J Med 2006;119:26–7.
4. Bouillet L, Launay D, Fain O, et al. Hereditary angioedema with C1inh deficiency: clinical presentation and quality of life of 193 French patients. Ann Allergy Asthma Immunol, in press.
5. Bouillet L, Longhurst H, Boccon-Gibod I, et al. Disease expression in women with hereditary angioedema. Am J Obstet Gynecol 2008;11:484.e1–4.
6. Yip J, Cunliffe WJ. Hormonally exacerbated hereditary angioedema. Australas J Dermatol 1992;33:35–8.
7. Bork K, Fischer B, Dewald G. Recurrent episodes of skin angioedema and severe attacks of abdominal pain induced by oral contraceptives or hormone replacement therapy. Am J Med 2003;114:294–8.
8. Borradori L, Marie O, Ryboad M, et al. Hereditary angioedema and oral contraception. Dermatologica 1990;181:78–9.
9. McGlinchey PG, McCluskey DR. Hereditary angioedema precipitated by estrogen replacement therapy in a menopausal woman. Am J Med Sci 2000;320: 212–3.
10. Saule C, Boccon-Gibod I, Fain O, et al. Benefits of progestin contraception in non-allergic angioedema. Clin Exp Allergy 2013;43:475–82.
11. Visy B, Füst G, Varga L, et al. Sex hormones in hereditary angioneurotic edema. Clin Endocrinol (Oxf) 2004;60:508–15.
12. Madeddu P, Emanueli C, Song Q, et al. Regulation of bradykinin B2 receptor expression by oestrogen. Br J Pharmacol 1997;121:1763–91.
13. Gordon EM, Douglas JG, Ratnoff OD, et al. The influence of estrogen and prolactin on Hageman factor (factor XII) titer in ovariectomized and hypophysectomised rats. Blood 1985;66:602–5.
14. Norris LA, Bonnar J. The effect of oestrogen dose and progestogen type on haemostatic changes in women taking low dose oral contraceptives. Br J Obstet Gynaecol 1996;103:261–7.
15. Gordon EM, Ratnoff OD, Saito H, et al. Rapid fibrinolysis, augmented Hageman factor (factor XII) titers, and decreased C1 esterase inhibitor titers in women taking oral contraceptives. J Lab Clin Med 1980;96:762–9.
16. Teede HJ, McGrath BP, Smolich JJ, et al. Postmenopausal hormone replacement therapy increases coagulation activity and fibrinolysis. Arterioscler Thromb Vasc Biol 2000;20:1404–9.

17. Nogawa N, Sumino H, Ichikawa S, et al. Effect of long term hormone replacement therapy on angiotensin converting enzyme activity and bradykinin in post menopausal women with essential hypertension and normotensive postmenopausal women. Menopause 2001;8:210–5.

18. Bork K, Wulff K, Hardt J, et al. Hereditary angiodema caused by missense mutations in the factor XII gene: clinical features, trigger factors, and therapy. J Allergy Clin Immunol 2009;124:129–34.

19. Vitrat-Hincky V, Gompel A, Dumestre-Perard C, et al. Type III Hereditary angiooedema: clinical and biological features in a French cohort. Allergy 2010;65: 1331–6.

20. Bork K, Barnstedt SE, Koch P, et al. Hereditary angioedema with normal C1-inhibitor activity in women. Lancet 2000;356:213–7, 27.

21. Binkley KE, Davis A. Clinical, biochemical, and genetic characterization of a novel estrogen-dependent inherited form of angioedema. J Allergy Clin Immunol 2000;106:546–50.

22. Martin L, Degenne D, Toutain A, et al. Hereditary angioedema type III: an additional French pedigree with autosomal dominant transmission. J Allergy Clin Immunol 2001;107:747–8.

23. Martin L, Raison-Peyron N, Nöthen MM, et al. Hereditary angioedema with normal C1 inhibitor gene in a family with affected women and men is associated with the p.Thr328Lys mutation in the F12 gene. J Allergy Clin Immunol 2007;120:975–7.

24. Bouillet L. Hereditary angioedema in women. Allergy Asthma Clin Immunol 2010; 6:17–20.

25. Martinez-Saguer I, Rusicke E, Aygören-Pürsün E, et al. Characterization of acute hereditary angioedema attacks during pregnancy and breast feeding and their treatment with C1 inhibitor concentrate. Am J Obstet Gynecol 2010;203: 131.e1–7.

26. Czaller I, Visy B, Csuka D, et al. The natural history of hereditary angioedema and the impact of treatment with human C1- inhibitor concentrate during pregnancy: a long term survey. Eur J Obstet Gynecol Reprod Biol 2010;152:44–9.

27. Picone O, Donnadieu AC, Brivet F, et al. Obstetrical complications and outcome in two families with hereditary angioedema due to mutation in the F12 gene. Obstet Gynecol Int 2010;2010:957507.

28. Caballero T, Farkas H, Bouillet L, et al. International consensus and practical guidelines on the gynecologic and obstetric management of female patients with hereditary angioedema caused by C1 inhibitor deficiency. J Allergy Clin Immunol 2012;129:308–20.

29. Bouillet L, Ponard D, Rousset H, et al. A case of hereditary angio-oedema type III presenting with C1-inhibitor cleavage and a missense mutation in the F12 gene. Br J Dermatol 2007;156:1063–5.

30. Lindoff C, Rybo G, Astedt B. Treatment with tranexamic acid during pregnancy, and the risk of thrombo-embolic complications. Thromb Haemost 1993;70: 238–40.

31. Baker JW, Craig TJ, Riedl MA, et al. Nanofiltered C1 esterase inhibitor (human) for hereditary angioedema attacks in pregnant women. Allergy Asthma Proc 2013; 34:162–9.

32. Farkas H, Csuka D, Tóth F, et al. Successful pregnancy outcome after treatment with C1-inhibitor concentrate in a patient with hereditary angioedema and a history of four miscarriages. Eur J Obstet Gynecol Reprod Biol 2012;165:366–7.

33. Rousset-Jablonski C, Thalabard JC, Gompel A. Tamoxifen contraindicated in women with hereditary angioedema? Ann Oncol 2009;20:1281–2.

34. Gelfand JA, Sherins RJ, Alling DW, et al. Treatment of hereditary angioedema with danazol. Reversal of clinical and biochemical abnormalities. N Engl J Med 1976; 295:1444–8.
35. Cicardi M, Castelli R, Zingale LC, et al. Side effects of long-term prophylaxis with attenuated androgens in hereditary angioedema: comparison of treated and untreated patients. J Allergy Clin Immunol 1997;99:194–6.
36. Zurlo JJ, Frank MM. The long-term safety of danazol in women with hereditary angioedema. Fertil Steril 1990;54:64–72.
37. Cicardi M, Bergamaschini L, Cugno M, et al. Long-term treatment of hereditary angioedema with attenuated androgens: a survey of a 13-year experience. J Allergy Clin Immunol 1991;87:768–73.

Contact System Activation in Patients with HAE and Normal C1 Inhibitor Function

Arije Ghannam, MD, PhD[a,b,1], Federica Defendi, PhD[a,b,1],
Delphine Charignon[a,b,1], Françoise Csopaki[b],
Bertrand Favier, DVM, PhD[a], Mohammed Habib, PhD[a],
Sven Cichon, PhD[c], Christian Drouet, PhD[a,b,*]

KEYWORDS

- Factor XII • Kallikrein • Kininogen • Kinin forming enzymes • Contact phase

KEY POINTS

- Contact phase proenzymes are activated in conditions when endothelium is triggered with diverse materials and under various conditions.
- The proenzyme to enzyme conversion is under the control by serpins, and proteolytic activity develops toward high-molecular-weight kininogen (HK).
- Hereditary angioedema with normal C1 inhibitor function (HAE-nC1INH) is associated with this biologic condition and, in a few cases (<10%), a missense mutation in the *F12* gene.

INTRODUCTION: NATURE OF THE PROBLEM

Kinin-mediated angioedema (AE) is a rare disorder characterized by recurrent and unpredictable episodes of localized swelling (face, extremities, bowel walls, genitals, and upper airways).[1,2] Occurring at the endothelium/plasma interface, this vascular permeability depends on the kinins (bradykinin [BK] and *des*Arg^9-BK) released on proteolytic enzymes on the precursor HK during activation of kallikrein (KK)-kinin system

Disclosure: The authors declare no competing financial interests. This work was supported by an ERA-Net E-RARE-1 research program within the framework of the project, Genetics, Pathophysiology, and Therapy of Hereditary Angioedema Type III (S. Cichon, coordinator).
[a] University Joseph Fourier, GREPI/AGIM CNRS FRE 3405, Grenoble, France; [b] French Reference Centre for Angioedema, CREAK, Grenoble, France; [c] Department of Genomics, Life & Brain Center, Institute of Human Genetics, University of Bonn, Germany and Division of Medical Genetics, Department of Biomedicine, University of Basel, Switzerland
[1] These authors contributed equally to this work.
* Corresponding author. University Joseph Fourier, GREPI/AGIM CNRS FRE 3405, CHU Grenoble, CS10217, Grenoble, F-38043 France.
E-mail address: christian.drouet@ujf-grenoble.fr

(alternatively described as contact system).[1–4] Plasma KK mainly supports the proteolytic activity toward HK.[5] With the renin-angiotensin system, the KK-kinin system represents the prototype of successful enzymatic mechanism elaborated during evolution for the control of vascular function. The enzyme components belong to the same chymotrypsin clan of serine proteases. Advancement in molecular enzymology and functional genomics brought to light a so-far unpredicted complexity of the vascular KK-kinin system and challenged the concept that the enzymatic component simply operates by accelerating a spontaneous biochemical reaction.

The important role for the KK-kinin system in hereditary angioedema (HAE) was revealed when it was found that fluids from blisters that were induced in HAE patients contained large amounts of KK, whereas similar blister fluids obtained from control individuals did not.[6] It is now established that inadequate control of the KK-kinin system activation and subsequent kinin overproduction give rise to HAE.[2,4,7] The diagnosis is classically based on the clinical picture in combination with the reduced C1 inhibitor (C1INH) function (<50%) associated or not with low levels of C1INH and C4.[8] Independent observations reported HAE-nC1INH manifesting as recurrent AE[9] without quantitative or functional C1INH abnormalities.[10,11] This form may be due to mutations in the *F12* gene (without thrombosis),[12,13] but in most cases the genetic basis remains to be determined. The authors previously demonstrated that in HAE-nC1INH the plasma of patients transiently develops an important increase of amidase activity (using the peptide substrate, PFR-pNA), which was initially qualified as a gain-of-function of factor XII (FXII).[12,14] The absence of a mutation in the *F12* gene in many patients raises the hypothesis that HAE-nC1INH actually is a heterogeneous condition.[15] HAE-nC1INH is currently diagnosed based on the observation of manifestations reminiscent of HAE and positive family history. The disease may often be underdiagnosed or overdiagnosed because of its nonspecific phenotype as well as variable severity and penetrance.

Evidence for KK-kinin system involvement in HAE-nC1INH comes from ex vivo studies that demonstrated its activation in plasma of patients,[12,15] and evidence for BK formation comes from successfully treatment with a B_2-receptor antagonist.[16] Because circulating kinins are short-lived peptides (27 $\pm$ 10 s) and circulate in very low concentrations (15–90 pM during attacks), however, evidence for the increased kinin production has indirectly been demonstrated by the cleavage of HK during the attacks.[17]

The burden of HAE-nC1INH and the efforts to properly diagnose the disease and to develop targeted treatment are substantial.[15] All the kinin-forming components are present in the plasma under the proenzyme state. The activation of kinin-forming proenzymes is initiated by FXII in a reaction involving HK and plasma prekallikrein (pKK) and under the C1INH control, collectively referred to as the plasma contact system.[18] The triggering mechanism of this pathway and the proenzyme activation process remain, however, poorly understood.

KININ-FORMING SYSTEM: COMPONENTS AND ACTIVATION PROCESS

The kinin-forming system is recent on the evolutionary scale: although a short BK containing protein is identified in jawless fish, the contact phase system (*pKK* and *F12* genes, together with a multidomain *HK* gene) appeared in some amniotes. All vertebrates and many nonvertebrate animals and arthropods, however, have a kinin-generating apparatus. This is consistent with the highly conserved development of inflammation and innate immunity between species. Moreover, it is remarkable that vascular endothelial and other cell types, including neutrophils and mast cells, express some or all members of the protein armamentarium with which to generate, degrade, and respond to endogenous kinins both in an autocrine and paracrine fashion. Given the short half-life of circulating kinins (a few seconds), it is not surprising that they are locally generated by injured/triggered tissues and that their physiologic and pathophysiologic actions are likely to be mediated on a local level.

On endothelial cells, HK assembles on a multiprotein receptor that consists of at least gC1qR, urokinase plasminogen activator receptor (u-PAR), and cytokeratin-1 (**Fig. 1**). Moreover, CK-1 colocalizes on endothelial cells with u-PAR but not gC1qR. HK is found primarily in plasma and some tissues. The majority of plasma pKK circulates in a complex with HK, a property shared with FXII. This allows HK bound to its multiprotein receptor to serve as the pKK receptor on endothelial cells.[19]

Components of the Kinin-forming System

In contrast to the kinin catabolism enzymes, which are spontaneously active in the plasma, the enzyme components of contact phase are present in the plasma as zymogens, which undergo enzyme conversion on activation conditions (discussed later). Terminology is summarized in **Table 1**.

High-molecular-weight kininogen

In mammalian species, there are 2 kininogens of different sizes, HK and low-molecular-weight kininogen (LK).[20] Synthesized in the liver, HK and LK are prototypes of modular plasma proteins that derive from differential RNA splicing of the single *KNG1* gene (11 exons).[21] They share the first N-terminal domains (D1–D3) and the BK D4 domain (see **Fig. 1A**). **Fig. 1B** shows the functional domains of HK interacting with its strategic partners: the N-terminal D1–D3 domains are homologous to cystatins but only the last 2 (D2 and D3) consist of specific sequences, QVVAG, that inhibit cysteine-proteases. D3 has platelet and endothelial cell-binding activity.[22] Adjacent to D3 is the KK-sensitive BK sequence (D4). At the C-terminal side of the BK moiety of HK, there are 2 unique domains (HK D5 and HK D6, the HK light chain [L chain]) that mediate contact phase activation.[21] Docking of HK to endothelium cell surface is stabilized by interactions between the His-rich sequence in the HK D5 domain and negatively charged sulfated proteoglycans on the cell surface[23] as well as by binding with CK-1.[24] With its pKK and factor XI–binding sites, HK D6 is responsible for the cofactor activity of HK in the plasma contact phase activation.[25,26]

HK circulates in plasma as an approximately 110-kDa single-chain glycoprotein at a concentration of 70 µg/mL to 90 µg/mL.[27]

Factor XII

FXII is an extraordinary protein because it links the KK-kinin system with the intrinsic coagulation cascade.[28] FXII is a serine protease produced by the liver that circulates in the blood as a single-chain under the zymogen form. The promoter of the *F12* gene has been shown to contain a functional estrogen-response element.[29] FXII consists of several structural domains: a fibronectin types II and I domain, 2 epidermal growth factor like (EGF-like) domains, a kringle domain, and a proline-rich region adjacent to its catalytic domain (**Fig. 2**). These domains are homologous to those found in other serine proteases, except the proline-rich region, which is unique to FXII.[30] FXII is highly susceptible to autoactivation after contact to negatively charged surfaces (eg, dextran sulfate, endotoxin, and heparin; **Table 2**) to become activated FXII (FXIIa) after a conformational change.[31] FXII can be also activated by KK: KK formation reciprocally activates more FXII in a reaction that is at least 1000-fold faster than autoactivation, with a reciprocal activation loop enhancing the rate of FXIIa and KK generation.

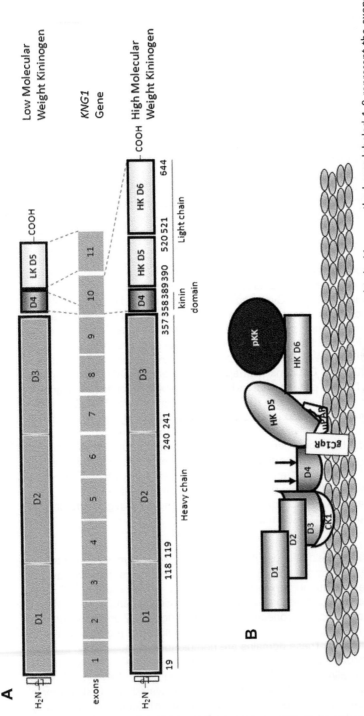

Fig. 1. (A) Diagrammatic representation of domains of HK and LK. The *KNG1* gene consists in 11 exons; the boxes labeled 1–9 represent the exons coding for H chain of both HK and LK. The gene uses alternative splicing to generate the 2 different proteins HK and LK. Exon 10 encodes the domain D4, which contains the BK sequence and both HK D5 and D6; exon 11 encodes the LK L chain (LK D5). The mature transcripts are assembled by the alternative splicing events in which the L-chain sequence is attached to the 3′-end of the 12-amino-acid common sequence, C-terminal relative to BK and with divergence of the HK and LK L-chain sequences at codon 402. LP, leader peptide. (*B*) HK functional domains. The H-chain region consists of 3 homologous domains D1–3, of which the latter 2 are cysteine protease inhibition sites. The HK-specific L-chain region contains the surface-binding sites (gC1qR and u-PAR; HK D5) and overlapping binding sites (cofactor) for pKK and factor XI (not illustrated; HK D6). The H and L chains are held together by a disulfide bond. Arrowheads indicate the sites of cleavage by plasma KK to release BK.

Table 1
Components of the kallikrein-kinin system

Current Name	Synonym	Abbreviation	Gene	Plasma Concentration
Kinin-forming proteases				
Factor XII	Hageman factor	FXII	*F12*	30–35 mg/L
Plasma prekalikrein	Fletcher factor	pKK	*KLKB1*	35–50 mg/L
Prolylcarboxypeptidase	—	PCP	—	—
Tissue kallikreins	—	tKK	*KLK1-15*	—
Kininogens				
High-molecular-weight kininogen	Fitzgerald trait (HK) and	HK	*KNG1*	70–90 mg/L
Low-molecular-weight kininogen	Flaugeac trait (HK + LK)	LK	*KNG1*	170–220 mg/L
Kinins				
Bradykinin	—	BK	—	—
*des*Arg^9-bradykinin	—	*des*Arg^9-BK	—	—
Lys-bradykinin	Kallidin	Lys-BK, KD	—	—
*des*Arg^{10}-kallidin	—	*des*Arg^{10}-KD	—	—
Kallikrein inhibitors				
C1 Inhibitor	—	C1INH	*SERPING1*	—
α_2-Macroglobulin	—	α_2-M	*A2M*	—
Kallistatin	—	—	*SERPINA4*	—
Kininases				
Angiotensin I–converting enzyme	Kininase II	ACE	*ACE*	—
Carboxypeptidase N	Kininase I	CPN	*CPN1, CPN2*	—
Carboxypeptidase M	—	CPM	*CPM*	—
Aminopeptidase P	—	APP	*XPNPEP2*	—
Dipeptidylpeptidase IV	CD26	DPPIV	*DPP4*	—
Neutral endopeptidase 24.11	CD10	NEP, CALLA, CD10	*MME*	—
Accessory participants				
u-Plasminogen activator receptor	—	u-PAR	*PLAUR*	—
Plasminogen	—	—	*PLG*	—
C1 proteases	—	C1r, C1s	*C1R, C1S*	—
Prolylcarboxypeptidase	—	PCP	*PRCP*	—
Kinin receptors				
B$_1$-receptor	—	B1R	*BDKRB1*	—
B$_2$-receptor	—	B2R	*BDKRB2*	—

Activation of FXII results in cleavage of the Arg_{353}-Val_{354} bond, generating an heavy chain (H chain) (353 residues) and an L chain (243 residues), held together by a disulfide bond. The H chain is responsible for binding to negatively charged surfaces, involving the positively charged amino acid sequence within residues 39–47 in the fibronectin type II domain (see **Fig. 2**); the L chain contains the catalytic domain. FXIIa can then activate pKK, C1 complex proenzymes (C1r and C1s), and FXI. FXIIa is a not able to directly cleave HK to produce BK. The FXIIa-driven contact system has proinflammatory and procoagulant activities via the KK-kinin system and the contact activation coagulation factor XI (FXI) pathway, respectively.

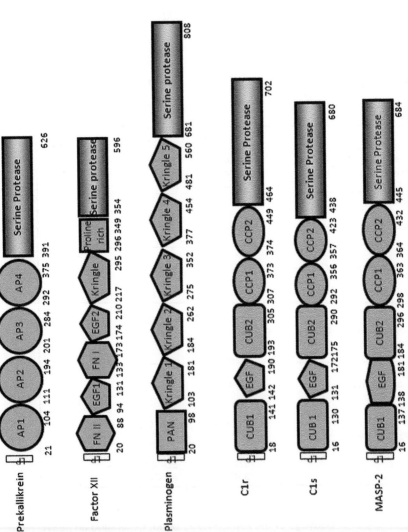

Fig. 2. Modular architecture of domains of pKK, FXII, plasminogen, C1r, C1s, and MASP-2. The 6 enzymes belong to the same chymotrypsin clan of serine proteases. The highly homologous catalytic domains of the serine proteases (SP domain) are located at the C-terminus. The N-terminal H chains comprise different modules specific to each protease: pKK with 4 AP modules; FXII with 2 FN modules, a Kringle module, and an electronegatively charged poly-Pro module; plasminogen with an N-terminal PAN module and 5 Kringle modules; complement C1r, C1s, and MASP-2 with an N-terminal CUB module, a Ca^{2+}-binding EGF-like module, a second CUB module, 2 CCP modules, and a chymotrypsin-like SP domain (nomenclature and symbols are as defined in Bork and Bairoch[91]). AP, Apple; CCP, Sushi (SCP); EGF, EGF-like; FN I/II, fibronectin type I or type II; LP, leader peptide; MASP, MBL Associated Serine Protease.

Table 2
Contact phase activators and their effects on inflammation and angioedema

Compound	In vitro Effect on Contact Phase	In vivo Effect	
		Proinflammatory	Angioedema
Nonphysiologic materials			
Glass beads	+	—	—
Kaolin	+	—	—
Ellagic acid	+	—	—
High-molecular-weight dextran sulfate	+	—	+
OSCS	+	—	+
Poly I:C	+	—	—
Carragheenan	+	+	+
Biomaterials	+	—	—
Dialysis membranes			
Cuprophan/polyacrylonitrile	+	+	+
Vascular grafts (Dacron/Polytetrafluoroethylene)	+	+	—
Metals			
Therapeutic compounds	+	?	?
Aptamers	+	?	?
Iron oxide nanoparticles	—	?	?
Endogenous substances			
Glycosaminoglycans	+	?	?
Nucleic acids (RNA, DNA)	+	?	?
Sulfatide (Gal sulfate sphingolipid)	+	+	?
Urate crystals	+	+	+
Misfolded protein aggregates	+	+	?
Amyloid-β peptide	+	+	?
Polyphosphates (60–100 residues)	+	+	+
Heparins	+	+	+
Chondroitin sulfate E	+	+	+
Bacterial lipopolysaccharide	+	+	+

Data from Maas C, Oschatz C, Renné T. The plasma contact system 2.0. Semin Thromb Hemost 2011;37:375–81.

Prekallikrein, plasma kallikrein, and tissue kallikreins

Two types of kallikreins (KKs) are responsible for the in vivo liberation of vasoactive kinins. These enzymes are genetically and structurally unrelated, but they both release kinins: (1) pKK is the zymogen of plasma KK, with HK as its main substrate, and is produced by the liver; (2) tissue KKs are a constitutively activated serine protease system (KK1 may be dominant), with LK as its main substrate, and originates from many cells (epithelial and endothelial cells, exocrine glandular cells, and neurons).

The pKK-encoding gene (*KLB1)* has significant homology to the gene coding for factor XI.[32] pKK binds to the C-terminal domain of HK (HK D6) and, through kininogen, the complex is bound on the surface of the vascular endothelium with high-affinity binding (Kd 15 nM) (**Fig. 3**). pKK is activated in KK during the contact phase[31,33]: FXIIa cleaves pKK at the scissile bond Arg_{371}-Ile_{372}, with subsequent production of the active KK with an H chain (371 residues) and an L chain (248 residues). The latter carries the catalytic domain (see **Fig. 2**).

Tissue KKs belong to a gene family comprising 15 genes (*KLK1*, the tissue KK1-encoding gene to *KLK15*).[34,35] KK1 is known to cleave efficiently LK, releasing

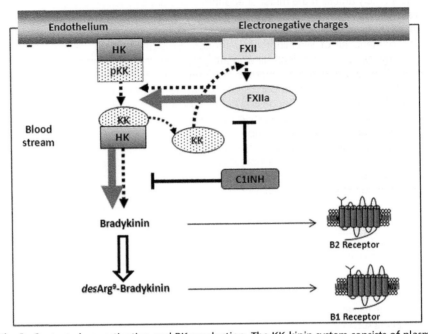

Fig. 3. Contact phase activation and BK production. The KK-kinin system consists of plasma proteins that assemble when blood comes into contact with triggers (eg, negatively charged surfaces): FXII, plasma pKK, and the nonenzymatic cofactor HK. Blood HK-pKK association (80%) is bound onto the endothelium. FXII and HK directly bind to polyanions, with subsequent putative conformational change in FXII leading to limited proteolytic activity. Consecutively, FXIIa cleaves pKK generating plasma KK. In an amplified reaction (*solid arrow*), KK efficiently activates further FXII zymogens and cleaves its cofactor HK to yield BK, the B_2-receptor ligand. Proenzyme activation and protease activities are under the C1INH control. HSP90 and PCP activate the pKK to KK conversion (*not shown*). Coagulation factor XI, the other substrate of FXII, has no role in BK formation and is not indicated in this scheme. The circulating carboxypeptidase N (CPN) converts BK into $desArg^9$-BK, the B_1-receptor ligand, and the membrane-bound (glycosyl-phosphatidylinositol anchor) aminopeptidase P (APP) and angiotensin I–converting enzyme (ACE) inactivate the receptor-binding capacity of both peptides. (*Data from* Defendi F, Charignon D, Csopaki F, et al. Actualités biologiques sur les angioedèmes à kinines. Rev Francoph Lab 2012;2012:39–52.)

Lys-BK, and to have a low affinity to HK. The natural substrates of the other tissue KKs are not well established. Tissue KK can probably produce kinins in the circulation near its secretion site and influence local blood flow before it becomes inactivated.

With cleavage by a KK, HK generates BK and LK generates Lys-BK (or kallidin). Although both BK and Lys-BK assume to activate the B_2-receptor with subsequent vasopermeation, the plasma KK with BK-generating capacity reflects on the major blood kinin-forming activity and is considered to mainly support the kininogenase activity responsible of the AE attacks.

Control by the serpins

Four serpins fully control the KK-kinin system activation and activity: C1INH, α_2-macroglobulin (α_2-M), α_2-antiplasmin (α_2-AP), and antithrombin III (ATIII), in order of importance. **Table 3** shows the relative serine protease control activities and predicts the relative effectiveness of the 4 main serpins. The control capacity of KK-kinin system is

Table 3
Control of contact phase, fibrinolysis, and complement proteases by serpins

Zymogen and Serpin	Plasma Concentration (μM)	Protease	Relative Effectiveness of Protease Control		Control by Serpins Ka ($M^{-1}s^{-1}$)	
					C1 Inhibitor	α_2-Macroglobulin
FXII	0.37	FXIIa	C1INH	91.3%	7.4×10^4	—
			α_2-AP	3.0%		
			ATIII	1.5%		
			α_2-M	4.3%		
pKK	0.4	Kallikrein	C1INH	52%	1.4×10^5	4.8×10^4
			α_2-M	35%		
			α_2-AP	8%		
			ATIII	1.1%		
C1s	0.3	C1s protease	C1INH	100%	4.3×10^5	—
C1r	0.3	C1r protease	C1INH	100%	4.1×10^4	—
MASP-2		MASP2	C1INH	100%	1.6×10^5 1.3×10^6 (heparin)	—
C1INH	1.7	—	—		—	—
α_2-M	3.6	—	—		—	—
α_2-AP	1.1	—	—		—	—
ATIII	2.6	—	—		—	—

Abbreviations: α_2-AP, α_2-antiplasmin; α_2-M, α_2-macroglobulin; ATIII, antithrombin III; MASP-2, MBL-associated serine protease 2.

performed under conditions of a serpin:protease molar excess (approximately 5:1) and a low binding affinity (k_{on} 1.4–41 $\times 10^4$ M^{-1} s^{-1}). Plasma concentrations of C1INH are most effective in inactivating KK (see **Table 3**). Sustained activation of the contact phase and complement, which can lead to depletion of C1INH, results in reduced control of FXII and KK. This decrease allows the reciprocal activation to proceed between these 2 proteases, resulting in sustained release of BK.

Tissue KK activity is under the control of the endogenous serpin kallistatin (serpin A4), a potent but nonexclusive inhibitor present in both blood and tissues with a slow serpin-protease complex forming kinetics[36] and KK-independent anti-inflammatory actions.[37]

Kallikrein-kinin System Activation

Activation process
As a largely established principle, the activation of the kinin system proceeds on electronegative surfaces. It involves a proenzyme to enzyme conversion, with getting hold of serine proteases exhibiting limited proteolytic activities to activate another zymogen and to cleave the HK substrate with subsequent BK production, so contact activation describes the unique property of FXII to undergo autoactivation and amplification with a putative change in shape when exposed to negatively charged surfaces. This assumption is strengthened by the low k_{on} values of the serine protease-serpin interactions (approximately 10^5 M^{-1} s^{-1}; see **Table 3**). The molecular basis for the formation of FXIIa remains, however, unknown. This process is likely to amplify fibrinolysis

and complement zymogens and vice versa (discussed later). Although many biologic substances allow for FXII autoactivation, their exposure to the zymogen does not occur constitutively in the intravascular compartment in nondisease states. This perception is particularly relevant for HAE-nC1INH patients where the amidase activity increases in plasma during the attack but keeps within the normal range through the interphase.[17]

On human umbilical vein endothelial cells, prolylcarboxypeptidase (PCP) has been identified as a pKK activator with serine protease properties and a K_M of 6.7 nM.[38] In addition, recent studies argue for direct effects of FXII on the protease-activated receptor (PAR3), which may contribute to contact system-driven platelet activation.

During activation of the pKK-HK complex on endothelial cells, BK is locally released from HK. FXIIa and plasmin also release kinins in vitro, but their importance in kinin formation in vivo is not established.

Contact phase activators

Nonphysiologic materials were the first substances described to activate contact phase; kaolin and celite are commonly used for coagulation diagnostics. The endothelial glycosaminoglycans are natural activators of FXII with BK production at the vessel wall.[23,39]

Aggregates of amyloid-β peptide initiate activation of KK-kinin system with production of BK in the cerebrospinal fluid of patients suffering from Alzheimer disease.[40] Platelets support FXII activation dependent on integrin αIIb-β3 signaling and enhance activation of the KK-kinin system in plasma.[41,42] On activation, platelets release from their dense granules various substances, including polyphosphates consisting of an inorganic linear polymer of phosphate units. Recent studies identified the platelet-derived polyphosphate responsible for FXII activation as a polymer of 60 to 100 phosphate residues. Platelet polyphosphate activates FXII in reconstituted systems and in plasma via direct binding, with subsequent FXIIa-dependent BK formation in vitro and in vivo.[43] High-molecular-weight dextran sulfate (500 kDa), a polysulfated polysaccharide of glucose moieties, is a potent stimulator of contact phase. Once injected in animals, it induces transient systemic BK-mediated hypotension; the drop of blood pressure is blocked by icatibant.[44] In 2007, lethal acute anaphylactoid hypotension affected patients receiving intravenous commercial heparin. A contaminant was identified in suspect preparations of heparin and characterized as non-natural occurring oversulfated chondroitin sulfate (OSCS).[45] OSCS activates contact phase and complement as potently as dextran sulfate and triggers KK-mediated BK formation in human plasma and in a model of experimental hypotonic shock in vivo.[46] Physiologic analogs (eg, mast cell chondroitin sulfates) have been proposed as activators of the contact phase in vitro.[47] The potency to contact-activate FXII decreases from dextran sulfate and OSCS (4 sulfate residues per disaccharide) to heparin (2.7 sulfate residues). Despite that the exact mechanism of proenzyme FXII activation is not known, BK-forming activity seems dependent on negative charge density of the polysaccharide rather than on a defined structure. **Table 2** gives an overview of the activators of contact phase.

Kinins are released under conditions of ischemia. Demonstration of increased kinin levels and possible protective effects of kinins during myocardial ischemia in the absence of ACE inhibitors support the contention that kinins may play a role in myocardial ischemia: in isolated normoxic rat hearts, kinins are released into the perfusate.[48] During ischemia, the respective kinin outflow increased more than 5-fold; thus, ischemia is a stimulus for an enhanced kinin release with contribution to reduce the sequelae of myocardial ischemia.[49]

In bacterial infection, bacterial endotoxins are released and can activate zymogens of the contact phase. Kinins are then produced in the systemic circulation and participate in septic shock.[50]

The KK-kinin system can also be activated by contact with artificial surface in extracorporeal circulations with subsequent kininformation and hypotension.[51]

Endothelium

The autoactivation process of FXII can include negatively charged surfaces (see **Table 2**). This activation along the endothelium requires zinc-dependent binding of FXII and HK to gC1qR, CK-1, and u-PAR. These 3 proteins complex together onto the cell membrane and the initiation depends on autoactivation of FXII upon binding to gC1qR. Activation of the contact system can also proceed on endothelial cell in the absence of FXII: in this instance, pKK activation depends on interaction with heat shock protein 90 (Hsp90)[52] or PCP.[38]

Neutrophil and mast cell

KK is a chemotactic factor for neutrophils[53]; it has been shown to cause neutrophil aggregation[54] and release of elastase.[55] FXIIa has also been shown to stimulate neutrophil aggregation and degranulation.[56] Neutrophils express B_1-receptor and the agonist stimulation of this receptor induces the neutrophil recruitment during inflammatory response[57]; desArg^9-BK, the B_1-receptor (B1R) ligand, increases endothelial production of chemokines, thereby facilitating the B1R-mediated neutrophil extravasation.[58] HK binding to neutrophils has been shown to depend on zinc concentration and MAC-1 (CD11b/CD18).[59]

Activated neutrophils and mast cells can secrete proteases with KK-like activity (eg, elastase that enables the formation of kinins,[60] tryptase that also could release kinins from both HK and LK in addition to activate pKK,[61] and neutrophil that secretes tissue KK).[62] In addition to histamine, mast cell secretory granules also contain highly sulfated polysaccharides with heparin as a major constituent. This glycosaminoglycan is synthesized exclusively by mast cells.[63] It has been identified as an FXII contact activator in vitro[47] and can initiate in vivo BK formation in an FXII-dependent manner.[64] This is consistent with the participation of the mast cell component in the BK-dependent vascular permeability.

INTERPLAY BETWEEN CONTACT PHASE, FIBRINOLYSIS, AND COMPLEMENT

Complement and the kinin system are closely linked in the endothelial permeability phenomenon.

In observation of AE patients, a production of plasmin is observed during the acute attacks.[65] FXII and KK activate plasminogen in plasma,[66] resulting in plasmin formation. Plasminogen activation by FXII may be due to the high homology of FXII and tissue plasminogen activator (tPA), a fibrinolysis initiator.[30] On cell surfaces, plasminogen activation is triggered by BK-stimulated release of tPA from endothelial cells.[67] u-PAR or urinary-type plasminogen activator can also activate plasminogen and can be of primary importance for its cell-mediated activation. In addition, the activation of fibrinolysis enhances kinin release by KK in inflammatory situations due to collaborative actions of plasmin and KK on HK.[68] The favorable effect of prophylactic treatment with tranexamic acid in patients with HAE (whatever the type of HAE) indicates that fibrinolysis activation could take place in BK production.[69] Tranexamic acid (4-[aminomethyl]cyclohexanecarboxylic acid) is a synthetic lysine derivative that forms a reversible complex with plasminogen at the lysine binding site. The reduction in plasminogen binding to fibrin seems to result in a decrease in the production of t-PA by endothelial cells or an increase in the rate of its clearance.

The contact phase has also the capacity to activate the complement classical[70,71] and alternative convertases.[72] Early work has shown that the rabbit ortholog of plasma KK is able to release the C5a as a result of a limited proteolysis of C5.[73] FXIIa has been demonstrated to activate complement C1 and subsequently the classical convertase.[71] In vitro, FXIIa triggers activation of the classical convertase and initiates the fibrinolysis via PK-mediated urokinase activation. On mast cells, C5a causes an upregulation of plasminogen activator inhibitor-1, which is able to neutralize the enzymatic activity of tPA.[74] Simultaneous activation of contact phase and complement often occurs in several pathologic conditions, including triggering conditions of AE. The actual control of these multiple protease systems by C1INH is also indicative of the close relationship between these proteolytic systems (see **Table 3**).[75] Evidence for interaction between complement and contact system is also supported by in vitro demonstration (using the Transwell model system) that the cytolytically inactive terminal complement complex induces the vascular leakage by the formation of BK and the release of platelet-activating factor.[76] It has also been shown that gC1qR, the receptor for the globular heads of C1q, specifically binds the HK L chain.[77] The molecular complex formed by gC1qR, u-PAR and CK-1 on the endothelial surface is able to bind pKK through HK and also binds FXII.

Fig. 4 shows the interconnections between the 3 proteolytic cascades.

PATIENT INVESTIGATIONS: GENETICS, BIOLOGIC PHENOTYPE, AND TESTING

HAE-nC1INH patients were formerly grouped under the name, idiopathic nonhistaminergic AE; this included both hereditary and sporadic forms; patients suffering from AE not prevented by anti-H1-histamine whose etiopathogenesis remains undefined.[78] The first familial observations reported clinical features indistinguishable from those of patients presenting with C1INH deficiency.[9,11,79] Frequently their AE was prevented by prophylaxis by tranexamic acid, a nonspecific antifibrinolytic drug likely to limit the amplification pathway dependent on plasmin.[69]

Table 4 shows the biologic characteristics of patients presenting with HAE-nC1INH. The plasma spontaneous amidase activity was assayed using the peptide substrate, H-D-Pro-Phe-Arg-pNA. The severity of disease depends on the kinin catabolism, mainly supported by aminopeptidase P, angioensin-I converting enzyme, carboxypeptidase N, and dipeptidylpeptidase IV.

Some light has been shed on etiopathogenic mechanisms that may underlay substantially idiopathic AE. Starting from evidence for linkage of the disease status with genetic markers on chromosome 5q in German and French kindreds, mutational analysis revealed a Thr328Lys mutation in the positional candidate gene *F12*.[12] In several other families, missense or deletion mutations in the *F12* gene segregated with the symptoms.[13,64,80–82] The Thr328Lys mutant was defined as a gain-of-function enzyme although it is still unexplained why the catalytic serine protease domain of the protease is untouched by the mutation. The additional electropositive charge in the polyproline domain of FXII could increase the susceptibility of proenzyme to activation; thus, gain-of-activation might be a more precise definition of the functional effect conferred by the FXIILys[328] protein. As an additional hypothesis, an escape of the mutant proenzyme to the control by C1INH could provide the FXIILys[328] protein with a functional benefit in the enzyme activation. A large majority of HAE-nC1INH situations are not associated with this mutant expression, and some patients exhibit a similar biologic phenotype, in favor of another protein mutant and in line of the observation of familial pedigrees.

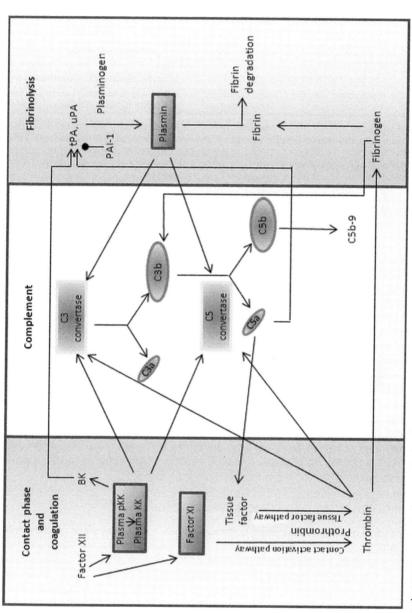

Fig. 4. Interplay between contact phase and complement. Components of the contact phase, fibrinolysis, and complement cascades develop positive interactions.

Table 4
Interpretation of patient data

Angioedema Type	Spontaneous Amidase Activity	Kinin Catabolism Enzymes
HAE-nC1Inh-F12c	↑ to ↑↑↑[a]	—
HAE-nC1Inh-F12nc[b]	↑ to ↑↑↑[a]	—
	—	↓ APP (OMIM[c] 300145) or ↓ ACE (OMIM[c] 106180) or ↓ CPN (OMIM 212070 and 603103) or ↓ DPPIV (OMIM[c] 102720)

Biologic investigation of HAE-nC1INH carrying or not the *F12* mutation (F12c and F12nc, respectively) is based on the measurements of plasma spontaneous amidase activity and the kinin catabolism.

Abbreviations: ACE, angiotensin I–converting enzyme; APP, aminopeptidase P; c, carrier; CPN, carboxypeptidase N; DPPIV, dipeptidylpeptidase IV; nc, noncarrier.

[a] During the AE attack.

[b] With the only biologic distinction by the C1INH function, failed kinin catabolism conditions and exaggerated kinin-forming activities overlap in the HAE-nC1INH entity.

[c] Online Mendelian Inheritance in Man (http://www.ncbi.nim.nih.gov/omim).

In some instances, the cleavage of C1INH was observed during the active periods of disease.[14] The cleavage was sustained during the pregnancy and C1INH function was found progressively decreased during pregnancy to nearly 50% at delivery, with important C1INH serpin cleavage without serpin-protease association.[64] The C1INH function returns to normal value out of the active period of disease. As a hypothesis, AE occurs in a context of uncontrolled proteolysis of C1INH serpin subsequent to the abundant contact phase proteases after activation of the Hageman factor mutant.

When patients present with an attack, plasma HK is transformed into the separated H and L chains, with or without the remnant native HK protein, as displayed by immunoblot with an anti–L-chain antibody.[83] The BK release during the attack can be appreciated from the abundance of the native HK compared with controls and the observation of the L-chain 46-kDa species gives evidence of the high protease input during the attacks (Bertrand Favier, DVM, PhD, personal communication, 2013). Complementary to HK analysis, the area under the curve of the kinetics of BK and *des*Arg^9-BK production in plasma on in vitro contact phase activation gives a more precise estimation of the kinin production during the attack.[84]

REPORTING, FOLLOW-UP, AND CLINICAL IMPLICATIONS

The absence of modified parameters commonly used in HAE diagnostic renders difficult the biologic diagnostic of HAE-nC1INH. In the absence of the identification of an *F12* gene mutation, the short-term increase of the plasma amidase activity in the periods of attacks is informative of the development of contact phase proteases and probably associated HK cleavage with BK production.[17] This transient kinin production in the AE condition is consistent with early observations where plasma, obtained from patients during an attack, strikingly increases vascular permeability in guinea pig skin, but samples obtained between attacks lack this property.[85]

As described previously, the HAE-nC1INH condition is commonly observed in female individuals. Because women were affected by this type of AE, the first descriptions referred the disease to as estrogen-dependent AE. Symptoms are actually precipitated by high estrogen levels, whether endogenous (pregnancy) or exogenous (oral contraceptives, hormone replacement therapy, or both) in origin.[11] This feature has been postulated to be associated with the estrogen-response element in the 5′ flanking region of the *F12* gene.[29] The level of plasma FXII was found normal, however, in affected female individuals. This condition of high AE frequency in female individuals coincides with the higher reference interval of the spontaneous amidase activity of female blood donors compared with that found in the male population (3.5 ratio).[17] The higher susceptibility of women and the triggering property of the estrogen input, however, remain unexplained.

Because of the rarity of the *F12* gene mutation within the families with HAE-nC1INH, the plasma amidase activity is useful for biologic testing.[14,86] It has been evaluated in patients presenting with HAE-nC1INH compared with HAE with C1INH deficiency, acquired angioedema, histamine-dependent AE, and anaphylaxis reactions. By fulfilling the conditions of the sampling in the period of attack, this assay may assist physicians and patients with meaningful argument. In complement to this assay, the evaluation of the HK cleavage and the kinetic parameters of the in vitro kinin production give evidence of the BK dependency of AE and an estimation of the BK production during the last hours.

OUTCOMES

Table 4 describes the distribution of AE etiopathologies in excessive kinin-production (including HAE with C1INH deficiency) and failed kinin catabolism. HAE-nC1INH can be recognized with these 2 conditions. Identification of families with failure of the kinin catabolism will contribute to distinguish between subgroups the HAE-nC1INH entity in the next future. In addition, independent etiopathogenesis conditions with both abnormalities of kinin formation and kinin catabolism can concur in situations related to HAE-nC1INH.[87] **Fig. 4** describes the activation of C3 convertases by KK, with subsequent anaphylatoxin production in line with the probable involvement in mast cell activation and the development of urticaria associated with HAE-nC1INH.[88]

CURRENT CONTROVERSIES/FUTURE CONSIDERATIONS

HAE-nC1INH seems to be a heterogeneous disease. As far as is known, mutations in the *F12* gene have been described as causative for some families with HAE-nC1INH and the presence of the SNP -2399A in the *XPNPEP2* gene as a possible aggravating factor.[81] In addition, low activity of plasma metallopeptidases of the kinin catabolism in HAE-nC1INH situations may give arguments for a responsibility of kininases in HAE-nC1INH. This leaves room for other gene mutations (in a monogenic sense) that could be involved in the development of HAE-nC1INH. Apart from this, the differences found in expressivity of the disease within families (also in families with *F12* mutations) leads the authors to postulate that the phenotype may be influenced by modifier genes.[82]

The question remains whether a proportion of disease cases might be multifactorial in origin. It could be speculated that inflammatory processes associated with kinins are related to infection conditions, where hosts can in principle use 2 different strategies to defend themselves against parasites: resistance and tolerance. Animals typically exhibit considerable genetic variation for resistance (ie, the ability to limit pathogen burden), when little is known about whether animals can evolve tolerance (ie, the ability to limit the damage caused by a given pathogen burden).[89,90] Considering the hypothesis that a certain proportion of AE cases might represent a multifactorial disease etiology, the pathologic load (ie, pathogen burden in the Råberg and his colleagues

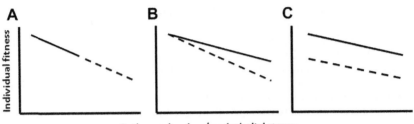

Fig. 5. Simplified scheme showing reaction norms of 2 individual genotypes (*dotted or solid line*) for disease severity across a range of pathologic burden in individuals. (*A*) Two equally tolerant genotypes differing in resistance; (*B*) two equally resistant genotypes (same average endothelial stress), but the genotype described with the dotted line is less tolerant; and (*C*) the genotypes differ in neither resistance (same average endothelial stress) nor tolerance (same slope). (*Data from* Råberg L, Sim D, Read AF. Disentangling genetic variation for resistance and tolerance to infectious diseases in animals. Science 2007;318:812–4.)

illustration) can be extended to endothelial stress as pathologic burden. Individuals suffering from AE might be distinguished between their capacities to develop resistance or tolerance to the AE trigger by 3 schemes (**Fig. 5**). In **Fig. 5**A, the genotype with the dotted line has lower endothelial stress (is more resistant) and thereby maintains a higher health status. In **Fig. 5**B, the genotype with the dotted line is less tolerant (health declines faster with increasing endothelial stress). In **Fig. 5**C, the gene difference exists even when the individuals are unstressed.

SUMMARY

Contact phase proenzymes are activated in conditions when endothelium is triggered with diverse materials and under various conditions. The proenzyme to enzyme conversion is under control by serpins, and proteolytic activity develops toward HK. HAE-nC1INH is associated with this biologic condition and, in a few cases, a mutation in the *F12* gene. Endothelium, mast cells, fibrinolysis, and complement participate in the triggering and the amplification of the process.

REFERENCES

1. Schapira M, Silver LD, Scott CF, et al. Prekallikrein activation and high-molecular-weight kininogen consumption in hereditary angioedema. N Engl J Med 1983;308:1050–3.
2. Björkqvist J, Sala-Cunill A, Renné T. Hereditary angioedema: a bradykinin-mediated swelling disorder. Thromb Haemost 2013;109:368–74.
3. Moreau ME, Garbacki N, Molinaro G, et al. The kallikrein-kinin system: current and future pharmacological targets. J Pharmacol Sci 2005;99:6–38.
4. Bas M, Adams V, Suvorava T, et al. Nonallergic angioedema: role of bradykinin. Allergy 2007;62:842–56.
5. Renné T, Gruber A. Plasma kallikrein: novel functions for an old protease. Thromb Haemost 2012;107:1012–3.
6. Curd JG, Prograis LJ Jr, Cochrane CG. Detection of active kallikrein in induced blister fluids of hereditary angioedema patients. J Exp Med 1980;152:742–7.
7. Cugno M, Zanichelli A, Foieni F, et al. C1-inhibitor deficiency and angioedema: molecular mechanisms and clinical progress. Trends Mol Med 2009;15:69–78.

8. Caballero T, Baeza ML, Cabañas R, et al. Consensus statement on the diagnosis, management, and treatment of angioedema mediated by bradykinin. Part I. Classification, epidemiology, pathophysiology, genetics, clinical symptoms, and diagnosis. J Investig Allergol Clin Immunol 2011;21:333–47 [quiz: 347].
9. Martin L, Degenne D, Toutain A, et al. Hereditary angioedema type III: an additional French pedigree with autosomal dominant transmission. J Allergy Clin Immunol 2001;107:747–8.
10. Bork K, Barnstedt SE, Koch P, et al. Hereditary angioedema with normal C1-inhibitor activity in women. Lancet 2000;356:213–7.
11. Binkley KE, Davis A 3rd. Clinical, biochemical, and genetic characterization of a novel estrogen-dependent inherited form of angioedema. J Allergy Clin Immunol 2000;106:546–50.
12. Cichon S, Martin L, Hennies HC, et al. Increased activity of coagulation factor XII (Hageman factor) causes hereditary angioedema type III. Am J Hum Genet 2006;79:1098–104.
13. Bork K. Hereditary angioedema with normal C1 inhibition. Curr Allergy Asthma Rep 2009;9:280–5.
14. Martin L, Raison-Peyron N, Nöthen MM, et al. Hereditary angioedema with normal C1 inhibitor gene in a family with affected women and men is associated with the p.Thr328Lys mutation in the F12 gene. J Allergy Clin Immunol 2007;120: 975–7.
15. Zuraw BL, Bork K, Binkley KE, et al. Hereditary angioedema with normal C1 inhibitor function: consensus of an international expert panel. Allergy Asthma Proc 2012;33(Suppl 1):S145–56.
16. Vitrat-Hincky V, Gompel A, Dumestre-Perard C, et al. Type III hereditary angiooedema: clinical and biological features in a French cohort. Allergy 2010;65: 1331–6.
17. Defendi F, Charignon D, Ghannam A, et al. Enzymatic assays for the biological diagnosis of bradykinin-dependent angioedema. PLoS One 2013;8: e70140.
18. Colman RW. Contact activation (Kallikrein-Kinin) pathway: multiple physiologic and pathophysiologic activities. In: Colman RW, Marder VJ, Clowes AW, et al, editors. Hemostasis and thrombosis. Basic principles and clinical practice. Philadelphia: Lippincott Williams & Wilkins; 2006. p. 109–13.
19. Shariat-Madar Z, Mahdi F, Schmaier AH. Factor XI assembly and activation on human umbilical vein endothelial cells in culture. Thromb Haemost 2001;85: 544–51.
20. Colman RW, Schmaier AH. The contact activation system: biochemistry and interactions of these surface-mediated defense reactions. Crit Rev Oncol Hematol 1986;5:57–85.
21. Kaufmann J, Haasemann M, Modrow S, et al. Structural dissection of the multidomain kininogens. Fine mapping of the target epitopes of antibodies interfering with their functional properties. J Biol Chem 1993;268:9079–91.
22. Jiang YP, Muller-Esterl W, Schmaier AH. Domain 3 of kininogens contains a cell-binding site and a site that modifies thrombin activation of platelets. J Biol Chem 1992;267:3712–7.
23. Renné T, Dedio J, David G, et al. High molecular weight kininogen utilizes heparan sulfate proteoglycans for accumulation on endothelial cells. J Biol Chem 2000;275:33688–96.
24. Shariat-Madar Z, Schmaier AH. Kininogen-cytokeratin 1 interactions in endothelial cell biology. Trends Cardiovasc Med 1999;9:238–44.

25. Tait JF, Fujikawa K. Primary structure requirements for the binding of human high molecular weight kininogen to plasma prekallikrein and factor XI. J Biol Chem 1987;262:11651–6.

26. Silverberg M, Nicoll JE, Kaplan AP. The mechanism by which the light chain of cleaved HMW-kininogen augments the activation of prekallikrein, factor XI and Hageman factor. Thromb Res 1980;20:173–89.

27. Adam A, Albert A, Calay G, et al. Human kininogens of low and high molecular mass: quantification by radioimmunoassay and determination of reference values. Clin Chem 1985;31:423–6.

28. Schmaier AH. The elusive physiologic role of Factor XII. J Clin Invest 2008;118:3006–9.

29. Farsetti A, Misiti S, Citarella F, et al. Molecular basis of estrogen regulation of Hageman factor XII gene expression. Endocrinology 1995;136:5076–83.

30. Stavrou E, Schmaier AH. Factor XII: what does it contribute to our understanding of the physiology and pathophysiology of hemostasis & thrombosis. Thromb Res 2010;125:210–5.

31. Samuel M, Pixley RA, Villanueva MA, et al. Human factor XII (Hageman factor) autoactivation by dextran sulfate. Circular dichroism, fluorescence, and ultraviolet difference spectroscopic studies. J Biol Chem 1992;267:19691–7.

32. Beaubien G, Rosinski-Chupin I, Mattei MG, et al. Gene structure and chromosomal localization of plasma kallikrein. Biochemistry 1991;30:1628–35.

33. Schmaier AH, McCrae KR. The plasma kallikrein-kinin system: its evolution from contact activation. J Thromb Haemost 2007;5:2323–9.

34. Clements JA, Willemsen NM, Myers SA, et al. The tissue kallikrein family of serine proteases: functional roles in human disease and potential as clinical biomarkers. Crit Rev Clin Lab Sci 2004;41:265–312.

35. Clements JA. Reflections on the tissue kallikrein and kallikrein-related peptidase family - from mice to men - what have we learnt in the last two decades? Biol Chem 2008;389:1447–54.

36. Zhou GX, Chao L, Chao J. Kallistatin: a novel human tissue kallikrein inhibitor. Purification, characterization, and reactive center sequence. J Biol Chem 1992;267:25873–80.

37. Yin H, Gao L, Shen Bo, et al. Kallistatin inhibits vascular inflammation by antagonizing tumor necrosis factor-alpha-induced nuclear factor kappaB activation. Hypertension 2010;56:260–7.

38. Shariat-Madar Z, Mahdi F, Schmaier AH. Identification and characterization of prolylcarboxypeptidase as an endothelial cell prekallikrein activator. J Biol Chem 2002;277:17962–9.

39. Renné T, Schuh K, Müller-Esterl W. Local bradykinin formation is controlled by glycosaminoglycans. J Immunol 2005;175:3377–85.

40. Bergamaschini L, Donarini C, Foddi C, et al. The region 1-11 of Alzheimer amyloid-beta is critical for activation of contact-kinin system. Neurobiol Aging 2001;22:63–9.

41. Castaldi PA, Larrieu MJ, Caen J. Availability of platelet factor 3 and activation of factor XII in thrombasthenia. Nature 1965;207:422–4.

42. Johne J, Blume C, Benz PM, et al. Platelets promote coagulation factor XII-mediated proteolytic cascade systems in plasma. Biol Chem 2006;387:173–8.

43. Müller F, Mutch NJ, Schenk WA, et al. Platelet polyphosphates are proinflammatory and procoagulant mediators in vivo. Cell 2009;139:1143–56.

44. Siebeck M, Cheronis JC, Fink E, et al. Dextran sulfate activates contact system and mediates arterial hypotension via B2 kinin receptors. J Appl Physiol 1994; 77:2675–80.

45. Guerrini M, Beccati D, Shriver Z, et al. Oversulfated chondroitin sulfate is a contaminant in heparin associated with adverse clinical events. Nat Biotechnol 2008;26:669–75.

46. Kishimoto TK, Viswanathan K, Ganguly T, et al. Contaminated heparin associated with adverse clinical events and activation of the contact system. N Engl J Med 2008;358:2457–67.

47. Hojima Y, Cochrane CG, Wiggins RC, et al. In vitro activation of the contact (Hageman factor) system of plasma by heparin and chondroitin sulfate E. Blood 1984;63:1453–9.

48. Baumgarten CR, Linz W, Kunkel G, et al. Ramiprilat increases bradykinin outflow from isolated hearts of rat. Br J Pharmacol 1993;108:293–5.

49. Lamontagne D, Nadeau R, Adam A. Effect of enalaprilat on bradykinin and des-Arg9-bradykinin release following reperfusion of the ischaemic rat heart. Br J Pharmacol 1995;115:476–8.

50. Cayla C, Todiras M, Iliescu R, et al. Mice deficient for both kinin receptors are normotensive and protected from endotoxin-induced hypotension. FASEB J 2007;21:1689–98.

51. Stoves J, Goode NP, Visvanathan R, et al. The bradykinin response and early hypotension at the introduction of continuous renal replacement therapy in the intensive care unit. Artif Organs 2001;25:1009–13.

52. Joseph K, Tholanikunnel BG, Kaplan AP. Heat shock protein 90 catalyzes activation of the prekallikrein-kininogen complex in the absence of factor XII. Proc Natl Acad Sci U S A 2002;99:896–900.

53. Kaplan AP, Kay AB, Austen KF. A prealbumin activator of prekallikrein. 3. Appearance of chemotactic activity for human neutrophils by the conversion of human prekallikrein to kallikrein. J Exp Med 1972;135:81–97.

54. Schapira M, Despland E, Scott CF, et al. Purified human plasma kallikrein aggregates human blood neutrophils. J Clin Invest 1982;69:1199–202.

55. Wachtfogel YT, Kucich U, James HL, et al. Human plasma kallikrein releases neutrophil elastase during blood coagulation. J Clin Invest 1983;72:1672–7.

56. Wachtfogel YT, Pixley RA, Kucich U, et al. Purified plasma factor XIIa aggregates human neutrophils and causes degranulation. Blood 1986;67: 1731–7.

57. Ehrenfeld P, Millan C, Matus CE, et al. Activation of kinin B1 receptors induces chemotaxis of human neutrophils. J Leukoc Biol 2006;80:117–24.

58. Duchene J, Lecomte F, Ahmed S, et al. A novel inflammatory pathway involved in leukocyte recruitment: role for the kinin B1 receptor and the chemokine CXCL5. J Immunol 2007;179:4849–56.

59. Wachtfogel YT, DeLa Cadena RA, Kunapuli SP, et al. High molecular weight kininogen binds to Mac-1 on neutrophils by its heavy chain (domain 3) and its light chain (domain 5). J Biol Chem 1994;269:19307–12.

60. Bhoola KD, Figueroa CD, Worthy K. Bioregulation of kinins: kallikreins, kininogens, and kininases. Pharmacol Rev 1992;44:1–80.

61. Imamura T, Dubin A, Moore W, et al. Induction of vascular permeability enhancement by human tryptase: dependence on activation of prekallikrein and direct release of bradykinin from kininogens. Lab Invest 1996;74:861–70.

62. Lauredo IT, Forteza RM, Botvinnikova Y, et al. Leukocytic cell sources of airway tissue kallikrein. Am J Physiol Lung Cell Mol Physiol 2004;286:L734–40.

63. Forsberg E, Pejler G, Ringvall M, et al. Abnormal mast cells in mice deficient in a heparin-synthesizing enzyme. Nature 1999;400:773–6.
64. Bouillet L, Ponard D, Rousset H, et al. A case of hereditary angio-oedema type III presenting with C1-inhibitor cleavage and a missense mutation in the F12 gene. Br J Dermatol 2007;156:1063–5.
65. Cugno M, Cicardi M, Agostoni A. Activation of the contact system and fibrinolysis in autoimmune acquired angioedema: a rationale for prophylactic use of tranexamic acid. J Allergy Clin Immunol 1994;93:870–6.
66. Kluft C, Trumpi-Kalshoven MM, Jie AF, et al. Factor XII-dependent fibrinolysis: a double function of plasma kallikrein and the occurrence of a previously undescribed factor XII- and kallikrein-dependent plasminogen proactivator. Thromb Haemost 1979;41:756–73.
67. Brown NJ, Gainer JV, Stein CM, et al. Bradykinin stimulates tissue plasminogen activator release in human vasculature. Hypertension 1999;33:1431–5.
68. Kleniewski J, Blankenship DT, Cardin AD, et al. Mechanism of enhanced kinin release from high molecular weight kininogen by plasma kallikrein after its exposure to plasmin. J Lab Clin Med 1992;120:129–39.
69. Du-Thanh A, Raison-Peyron N, Drouet C, et al. Efficacy of tranexamic acid in sporadic idiopathic bradykinin angioedema. Allergy 2010;65:793–5.
70. Ghebrehiwet B, Silverberg M, Kaplan AP. Activation of the classical pathway of complement by Hageman factor fragment. J Exp Med 1981;153:665–76.
71. Ghebrehiwet B, Randazzo BP, Dunn JT, et al. Mechanisms of activation of the classical pathway of complement by Hageman factor fragment. J Clin Invest 1983;71:1450–6.
72. Discipio RG. The activation of the alternative pathway C3 convertase by human plasma kallikrein. Immunology 1982;45:587–95.
73. Wiggins RC, Giclas PC, Henson PM. Chemotactic activity generated from the fifth component of complement by plasma kallikrein of the rabbit. J Exp Med 1981;153:1391–404.
74. Wojta J, Kaun C, Zorn G, et al. C5a stimulates production of plasminogen activator inhibitor-1 in human mast cells and basophils. Blood 2002;100:517–23.
75. Davis AE III. The pathophysiology of hereditary angioedema. Clin Immunol 2005;114:3–9.
76. Bossi F, Fischetti F, Pellis V, et al. Platelet-activating factor and kinin-dependent vascular leakage as a novel functional activity of the soluble terminal complement complex. J Immunol 2004;173:6921–7.
77. Joseph K, Ghebrehiwet B, Kaplan AP. Cytokeratin 1 and gC1qR mediate high molecular weight kininogen binding to endothelial cells. Clin Immunol 1999;92:246–55.
78. Cicardi M, Bergamaschini L, Zingale LC, et al. Idiopathic nonhistaminergic angioedema. Am J Med 1999;106:650–4.
79. Bork K, Siedlecki K, Bosch S, et al. Asphyxiation by laryngeal edema in patients with hereditary angioedema. Mayo Clin Proc 2000;75:349–54.
80. Dewald G, Bork K. Missense mutations in the coagulation factor XII (Hageman factor) gene in hereditary angioedema with normal C1 inhibitor. Biochem Biophys Res Commun 2006;343:1286–9.
81. Duan QL, Binkley K, Rouleau GA. Genetic analysis of Factor XII and bradykinin catabolic enzymes in a family with estrogen-dependent inherited angioedema. J Allergy Clin Immunol 2009;123:906–10.

82. Gómez-Traseira C, López-Lera A, Drouet C, et al. Hereditary angioedema caused by the p.Thr309Lys mutation in the F12 gene: a multifactorial disease. J Allergy Clin Immunol, in press.
83. Hentges F, Hilger C, Kohnen M, et al. Angioedema and estrogen-dependent angioedema with activation of the contact system. J Allergy Clin Immunol 2009; 123:262–4.
84. Ghannam A, Luyasu S, Drouet C. Diagnostic et traitement de l'angioedème. EP1153239 (2011).
85. Donaldson VH, Ratnoff OD, Dias Da Silva W, et al. Permeability-increasing activity in hereditary angioneurotic edema plasma. II. Mechanism of formation and partial characterization. J Clin Invest 1969;48:642–53.
86. Bergmann MM, Caubet JC, Defendi F, et al. Oestrogen-independent hereditary angioedema with normal C1 inhibitor function in a 10-year-old boy. Ann Allergy Asthma Immunol 2013;11:67–9.
87. Guichon C, Floccard B, Coppéré B, et al. One hypovolaemic shock…two kinin pathway abnormalities. Intensive Care Med 2011;37:1227–8.
88. Giard C, Nicolie B, Drouet M, et al. Angio-oedema induced by oestrogen contraceptives is mediated by bradykinin and is frequently associated with urticaria. Dermatology 2012;225:62–9.
89. Råberg L, Sim D, Read AF. Disentangling genetic variation for resistance and tolerance to infectious diseases in animals. Science 2007;318:812–4.
90. Maas C, Oschatz C, Renné T. The plasma contact system 2.0. Semin Thromb Hemost 2011;37:375–81.
91. Bork P, Bairoch A. Extracellular protein modules: a proposed nomenclature. Trends Biochem Sci 1995;20.

Role of the B1 Bradykinin Receptor and gC1qR/p33 in Angioedema

Fleur Bossi, PhD[a,b,*], Francesco Tedesco, MD[a]

KEYWORDS

- Angioedema • Vascular leakage • gC1qR/p33 • BK 1 receptor • BK 2 receptor

KEY POINTS

- The features and signs seen in angioedema (AE) lesions are typical of the inflammatory process, but increased vascular permeability predominates, leading to dermal and subcutaneous edema.
- gC1qR/p33 may represent a natural surface receptor that modulates or triggers the coagulation/kinin cascade, causing the generation of bradykinin (BK) and related kinins.
- Both B1 and B2 BK receptors are involved in AE episodes.
- Experimental data suggest that the blockade of both B1 and B2 receptors, or gC1q/p33, may provide novel therapeutic targets to induce symptom relief.

CLINICAL FEATURES OF ANGIOEDEMA EPISODES

Patients affected by angioedema (AE) are subject to asymmetric, nonerythematous, nonpruritic, localized, transient, episodic swelling of deeper layers of the skin or submucosal tissues of the skin, oropharyngolaryngeal tissue, and/or gastrointestinal wall (**Fig. 1**).[1] When the swelling occurs in the intestine, it causes severe abdominal pain, reminiscent of appendicitis, and intestinal obstructions. When the colon is affected, severe watery diarrhea may occur. Swelling in the larynx is the most dangerous symptom, because the affected individual may suffocate. The features and signs seen in AE lesions are typical of the inflammatory process but increased vascular permeability predominates, leading to massive dermal and subcutaneous edema, becoming

Disclosure: The authors have no relationship with a commercial company that has a direct financial interest in the subject matter or materials discussed in the article or with a company making a competing product.

[a] Department of Life Sciences, University of Trieste, via Valerio 28, Trieste 34127, Italy;
[b] Department of Medical, Surgical and Health Sciences, University of Trieste, Strada di Fiume 447, Trieste 34149, Italy
* Corresponding author. Department of Medical, Surgical and Health Sciences, University of Trieste, Strada di Fiume 447, Trieste 34149, Italy.
E-mail address: fbossi@units.it

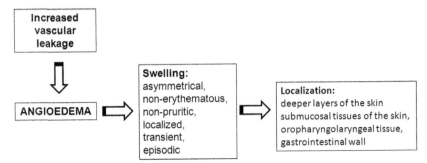

Fig. 1. Clinical signs of angioedema episodes.

particularly life threatening if it occurs in the upper respiratory tract. AE affects at least 20% of the population and several forms recur chronically, causing significant personal, domestic, social, and occupational disability.

Different forms of AE can be distinguished based on the presence or absence of chronic recurrence or significant urticaria. Acute AE is frequently a direct consequence of exposure to a specific substance (usually a food, chemical, or drug) eliciting an allergic/pseudoallergic reaction, which releases histamine. Chronic recurrent AE, occurring with prominent urticarial flare, is typically histamine mediated. More mysterious is the condition of chronically recurrent AE without urticaria. Such episodes may be triggered by trauma, menstrual periods, excessive exercise, or exposure to extremes of temperature or mental stress, but most events remain apparently spontaneous.[2,3] This situation is frequently seen in cases of inherited C1 inhibitor (C1-INH) deficiency and in AE related to angiotensin-converting enzyme (ACE) inhibitor treatment. AE associated with C1-INH deficiency is an inherited (hereditary angioneurotic edema [HAE]) or acquired (acquired angioedema) clinical condition that affects approximately 1:50,000 subjects in the general population.[4,5] The inherited deficiency is caused by mutations in the C1-INH gene, whereas the acquired form is the result of protein hypercatabolism, frequently caused by autoantibodies to C1-INH, and is associated with lymphoproliferative disorders and, in a few instances, with solid neoplasia, autoimmune, and infectious diseases.[6–8] Although the pathogenesis of the swelling associated with HAE was originally thought to be mediated by complement and, more specifically, by C2-derived kinin, evidence now exists that the swelling involves primarily the kinin-forming pathway.[3,9]

In spite of a lifelong stable C1-INH deficiency or continuous ACE inhibitor treatment, patients with these conditions are only seldom symptomatic, with huge variation in frequency and severity of symptoms. The mechanism(s) responsible for such variability is unexplained and, despite the progress that has been made in recent years, the molecular mechanisms underlying AE, particularly in the chronic forms, are still largely unknown. To unravel the pathogenesis of AE, the molecular players should be identified, including the factors that act to localize the event at a specific site, the mediator(s) that induce permeability on the vascular structures, and the enzymatic systems promoting the release of such mediator(s). The increase of vascular permeability may be induced by different factors. Histamine is the best characterized mediator that causes the vascular response. However, several systems may be activated during AE attacks, and the contact system, the factor XII (FXII)–dependent fibrinolytic cascade, and the complement system seem to be the most important factors involved in the disease.[10]

Available evidence suggests that the nonapeptide bradykinin (BK), generated at the endothelial cell surface, may be largely responsible for the vascular permeability seen in most AE, which does not respond to antihistamine. This possibility is supported by the presence of high levels of BK in the plasma of patients during acute attacks but not when in remission. Patients with AE that is responsive to antihistamines do not have increased levels of BK even during acute attacks. These data suggest the existence of 2 distinct groups of AE: histaminergic and nonhistaminergic. Histaminergic AE responds to antihistamines, whereas nonhistaminergic AE is more difficult to treat. In these cases the treatment of AE attacks involves drugs that function as BK B2 receptor antagonists (icatibant/HOE-140) or restore the control of BK formation through the inhibition of kallikrein (Dx88 and plasma-derived C1-INH). The result of the treatment is rapid relief, but complete resolution of symptoms is rarely obtained in less than 12 hours.[11]

ROLE OF GC1QR IN BK RELEASE ON EC

Because simultaneous and unregulated activation of both the complement (C) and kallikrein-kinin systems on the endothelial surface is largely responsible for the BK-mediated vascular permeability leading to edema, identification and characterization of the molecule or molecules that facilitate the assembly and activation of the kinin-generating pathway have been the focus of intense research over the past 20 years.

The ECs are activated by the late C components from C5 to C9 that form the terminal C complex (TCC). The formation of this complex is initiated with the release of C5b from cleaved C5, followed by progressive binding of the remaining late C components from C6 to C9. This complex may cause cytolysis through a pore formation following insertion into the plasma membrane of target cells,[12] or as a sublytic complex that fails to cause cell lysis despite its binding to the phospholipids bilayer of the cell membrane. The TCC can also assemble in the fluid phase, where it accumulates as a cytolytically inactive complex because of the short half-life of its cell-binding ability. The complex binds the soluble C regulators S protein and clusterin and circulates in plasma or is present in the extravascular fluid as SC5b-9.[13] We have shown that this complex, despite its inability to cause cytolysis, promotes vascular leakage.[13] This effect was documented in vitro using a Transwell system to evaluate the leakage of fluorescein-labeled bovine serum albumen (BSA) or the intravital microscopy to follow the extravasation of circulating FITC-BSA across mesenteric microvessels.[13] The permeabilizing activity of SC5b-9 was partially inhibited by the B2R antagonist (HOE-140), or the selective platelet activating factor (PAF) receptor antagonist (CV3988) and was completely neutralized by the mixture of the two antagonists, suggesting that the effect of SC5b-9 is mediated by the formation of BK and the release of PAF.

Our observation was further supported by the finding of high levels of SC5b-9 in pleural fluids of patients affected by Dengue virus infections.[14] In these patients, who die mainly from vascular leakage and shock, the nonstructural viral protein 1 (NS1) activates C, resulting in the release of anaphylotoxins and SC5b-9. The plasma levels of NS1 and SC5b-9 correlated with the disease severity, suggesting that the anaphylotoxins and the terminal complex may contribute to the pathogenesis of the vascular permeability. A significant activation of the terminal pathway of the C sequence was also observed during the attack phase of hereditary AE, as documented by the increased levels of SC5b-9 measured in patients during the attack phase.[15] These data, together with the in vitro and in vivo observations indicating a clear permeabilizing activity of SC5b-9,[13] suggest the existence of a crosstalk between the C and the kinin systems in induction of vascular leakage during the acute episodes of AE.

To date, 3 endothelial cell–binding sites for high-molecular-weight kininogen (HK) and FXII have been described. These sites include the 33-kDa cell surface receptor for the first component of C C1q (gC1qR/p33),[16–18] cytokeratin 1,[19,20] and the urokinase plasminogen activator receptor (uPAR) (**Fig. 2**).[21] Although the 3 proteins bind HK and/or FXII in a zinc-dependent manner and are postulated to form a multiprotein receptor complex with each contributing to the recruitment and assembly of the kinin-generating pathway proteins,[22] gC1qR/p33, which binds specifically to domain 5 in the light chain of HK,[18,23] may play a central role by virtue of its high affinity for HK. Although HK binds to isolated gC1qR/p33 with a dissociation constant (K_d) of 0.8 ± 0.7 nM (on-rate constant [k_{on}] = $12.3 \pm 5.0 \times 10^4$ $M^{-1}s^{-1}$; off-rate constant [k_{off}] = $0.8 \pm 0.5 \times 10^{-4}$ $M^{-1}s^{-1}$),[24] the binding of HK to gC1qR expressed on endothelial cell surface is 9 ± 2 nM. This binding is completely inhibited by mAb 74.5.2, which recognizes the C-terminal half of gC1qR/p33 corresponding with residues 204 to 218.[17,25] In contrast, domain 5 of HK, located at the N-terminus of the light chain, is rich in histidine and arginine residues and contains the site for interaction with gC1qR/p33. A 20 amino acid peptide corresponding with domain 5 and termed HKH20 has been synthesized and shown to inhibit the interaction of HK with intact endothelial cells.[18,23]

gC1qR/p33, uPAR, and CK-1, which are present on the EC surface, are able to bind the molecular complex formed by prekallikrein (PK), HK, and FXII (see **Fig. 2**).[26,27] Following this interaction, a serine protease (prolylcarboxypeptidase [PRCP]), expressed on the cell membrane, cleaves PK.[28] The activated kallikrein modifies FXII, leading to its activation, which in turn can increase the kallikrein formation on ECs. The main substrate of kallikrein is HK, which releases the vasoactive peptide BK.[26] These data suggest that gC1qR/p33 may represent a natural surface receptor that modulates or triggers the coagulation/kinin cascade, causing the generation of the potent proinflammatory peptide BK and related kinins (Lys-BK, des-Arg^9-BK, Lys-des-Arg^9-BK).

BK can also be generated through another pathway that starts intracellularly. First, conversion of prekallikrein to tissue kallikrein takes place inside the cell and the kallikrein generated in this manner is then secreted into the pericellular milieu. Second, the secreted kallikrein digests low-molecular-weight kininogen (LK) to generate the decapeptide, lysyl-BK (Lys^0-BK) or kallidin.[29,30] Third, kallidin is converted to the nonapeptide BK by the zinc-dependent enzyme called aminopeptidase.[31] BK produced by either pathway is then degraded in a sequential manner to lower-molecular-weight peptides by 3 kininases including carboxypeptidase N, ACE, and aminopeptidase P.[31–33] The major plasma enzyme is carboxypeptidase N, which removes the C-terminal arginine from BK to yield an octapeptide, des-arg^9-BK (**Fig. 3**).[32,33] The

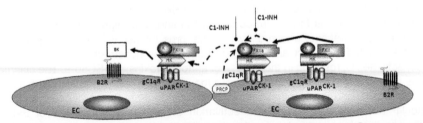

Fig. 2. Role of gC1qr/p33 in angioedema episodes. The molecules factor XII (FXII), prekallikrein (PK), and HK interact with the endothelial cell membrane through a binding site formed by gC1qR/p33, urokinase plasminogen activator receptor (uPAR), and cytokeratin 1 (CK-1). The consequent activation of kallikrein (K) by FXIIa and prolylcarboxypeptidase (PRCP) leads to the generation of BK that can stimulate the B2R.

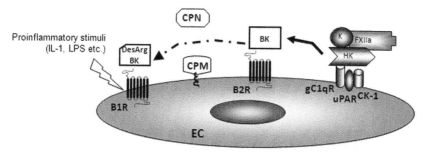

Fig. 3. Role of bradykinin receptors in angioedema episodes. BK released from the activation of the kinin system along the endothelial cell surface can interact with B2 receptors or can be cleaved by carboxypeptidase M (CPM), on the cell membrane, or CPN, in soluble phase, forming des-Arg9-BK, which is the agonist for B1R, membrane expression of which is induced by proinflammatory molecules.

second kininase in plasma is kininase II, which is identical to ACE and is found mainly along the pulmonary vascular endothelial cell surface. This kininase removes the dipeptide phe-arg from the C-terminus of BK to yield a heptapeptide, and a second cleavage removes ser-pro to leave a pentapeptide.[34]

The release of BK may be controlled by C1-INH, which belongs to a family of serine protease inhibitors called serpins, which together constitute 20% of all plasma proteins.[1] This serpin is a glycoprotein of 478 amino acid residues encoded by a single-copy gene on chromosome 11 and synthesized by the liver, fibroblasts, monocytes, macrophages, ECs, and other cell types.[35] C1-INH is the sole known inhibitor of C1r and C1s proteases of the first C component (C1), and moreover inactivates the complex formed by mannose binding protein and mannose-associated serine proteases,[36] and inhibits the alternative pathway.[37] In addition, C1-INH is able to control the serine proteases of the clotting and the kinin systems, including FXIIa and factor XIa, kallikrein, plasmin, and tissue plasminogen activator, which are activated by injury to blood vessels and by some bacterial toxins.[35] C1-INH deficiency leads to the onset of AE. Nevertheless, the possibility that activation of both the complement and the kinin-forming systems may contribute to the edema has not been completely excluded. Activated plasma kallikrein, with the contribution of FXII, initiates the kinin cascade (see **Fig. 2**), cleaving HK to generate BK. Nussberger and colleagues[38] documented that levels of BK were increased in the plasma of patients with AE. FXIIa is also capable of activating C1 and plasmin, leading to the cleavage of C2 into a kininlike fragment (C2 kinin).[39] BK, and possibly this fragment, can cause enhanced postcapillary venule permeability, presumably mediated by B1R and B2R localized on the endothelial cell membrane.[40] This mechanism is responsible for the edema and movement of fluid from the vascular space into the tissues.

We recently used both in vitro and in vivo permeability assays to analyze the ability of plasma collected during the attack phase plasma (APL) from C1-INH–deficient patients to cause endothelial leakage.[41] Using human adult dermal microvascular ECs and ECs isolated from the human umbilical vein, we were able to show that APL induced a delayed FITC-BSA leakage (30 minutes) as opposed to the rapid effect of BK (5 minutes), whereas remission plasma (RPL) elicited a modest effect compared with the control plasma. These data were also confirmed by in vivo experiments using intravascular microscopy. APL, RPL, and BK were administered via topical application on rat mesenteric microvessels. APL induced a significant increase in vascular leakage, whereas RPL had no effect. Incubation of cultured endothelial cells with a monoclonal antibody against the gC1qR/p33 abrogated the permeabilizing effect of APL observed in the in vitro model.

ROLE OF BK RECEPTORS

BK is a powerful endothelium-dependent peptide that, in addition to its well-known function in vasodilation, enhancement of vascular permeability, and smooth muscle constriction, has also been implicated in various pathophysiologic processes including hypotension, tumor angiogenesis and metastasis, and pain.[30,42] More importantly, BK is thought to play a critical role in the onset of the rare disease HAE. BK action and signaling are mediated by two 7-transmembrane domain–containing G-protein–coupled receptors named B1 receptor (B1R) and B2R. Although the B2R is ubiquitously and constitutively expressed in healthy tissues, B1R is induced and synthesized de novo as a consequence of tissue injury or inflammation (see **Fig. 3**).[40,43] Furthermore, although the B2R displays high affinity for BK and Lys-BK peptide agonists, the B1 receptor displays highest affinity to des-Arg^9-BK and des-Arg^9-kallidin. Following initial stimulation of B2 receptors, the action of BK is further enhanced by secondary production of vasodilators such as nitric oxide (NO), and prostacyclins, which exacerbate the inflammatory process.[40,42] An undesired side effect of ACE inhibitors, a class of drugs used to treat patients with hypertension and congestive heart failure, is the inhibition of BK degradation. This in turn increases plasma levels of BK, thereby causing hypotension and vascular permeability.[40,43]

The release of BK and related peptides and their interaction with B1R or B2R often lead to pathologic conditions usually characterized by increased vascular permeability. Increased retinal vascular permeability can be caused by loss of retinal endothelial tight junctions. This disorder is mediated by the carbonic anhydrase-I–induced alkalinization of the corpus vitreum, which promotes the enzymatic activity of kallikrein and the generation of activated FXII. This activation promotes the formation of kinins, which are eventually responsible for increase of vascular leakage.[44] The same permeabilizing effect of kinins released after stimulation by carbonic anhydrase-I is presumably responsible for intracerebral hemorrhage and edema.[44] Experimental evidence underlines that the role of B2R is more important than that of B1R in the blood-brain disruption and brain edema in ischemic stroke.[45] However, the relevant contribution of B1R has been shown in other pathologic conditions such as endotoxic shock[46] and maintenance of intra-articular edema in arthritis.[47] B1R and B2R are also involved in the vascular leakage seen in tumors and infections. In particular, antagonists of B2R are able to suppress vascular permeability in solid tumors and reduce accumulation of ascitic fluid.[48] Bacterial surfaces can directly activate HK leading to the release of BK, which in turn can be transformed by bacterial proteases to B1 agonists and in this way contribute to bacterial dissemination.[48]

The involvement of B2R in the onset of HAE symptoms is supported by the ameliorative effect obtained treating the patients with HOE-140 (icatibant), a selective antagonist of B2R.[49] However, despite the immediate relief obtained with this drug, complete resolution of symptoms requires several hours, raising the hypothesis that other molecules and receptors are involved in the maintenance of AE.

Using both in vitro and in vivo models, we have shown that HOE-140 induced a partial reduction of APL-induced BSA leakage, as did either of the two B1R antagonists (R715 and R954), whereas combined treatment with B1R and B2R antagonists completely inhibited the leakage. Because B2R is constitutively expressed but B1R expression is induced by proinflammatory stimuli such as IL-1β, we treated ECs first with IL-1β and then with APL from patients with inherited or acquired AE. That treatment induced a further increase of vascular leakage. To further evaluate the role of B1R, brefeldin A, which is a protein trafficking inhibitor, was used, and that treatment was able to reduce the permeabilizing effect of the APL.[41] These data suggest that the interaction between the HK-prekallikren-FXII molecular complex and gC1qR/p33, which leads to the formation of BK and des-Arg9-BK, and B1R expression represent critical steps in the development of AE and that blockade of both B1R and B2R receptors, or gC1q/p33, may provide novel therapeutic tools to better control the symptoms of the acute attack in patients with AE.

SUMMARY

From experimental evidence reported in this article, it is evident that both the kinin and the complement systems are involved in pathologic conditions characterized by increased vascular permeability. These two systems closely cooperate and their interplay between the complement and the kinin systems is established at different levels: the vascular leakage induced by SC5b-9 is mediated by PAF and BK; the essential role played by C1-INH in controlling both the activation of the complement cascade and many of the serine proteases involved in the clotting and kinin formation processes; the presence of gC1qR/p33 onto the EC surface, where it functions as a receptor for the molecular complex HK-PK-FXII leading to the release of BK. All these events indicate that there is a crosstalk between the complement and the kinin systems, and all the activation products coming from both these pathways have a common target: the endothelium. During the AE attacks, the deficiency of C1-INH results in the activation of the serine proteases, leading to the release of BK through the interaction between HK-PK-FXII and gC1qR/p33. Enzymes expressed on the EC membrane can metabolize BK producing the agonist of the B1R, which can then be upregulated by proinflammatory stimuli such as IL-1β. These data suggest that the blockade of both B1R and B2R, or gC1q/p33, may provide novel therapeutic targets to induce symptom relief.

REFERENCES

1. Beltrani VS. Angioedema: some new thoughts regarding idiopathic angioedema. In: Greaves MV, Kaplan AP, editors. Urticaria and angioedema. New York: Marcel Dekker; 2004. p. 421–39.
2. Davis AE 3rd. The pathophysiology of hereditary angioedema. Clin Immunol 2005;114:3–9.
3. Kaplan AP. C1 inhibitor deficiency. In: Greaves MV, Kaplan AP, editors. Urticaria and angioedema. New York: Marcel Dekker; 2004. p. 303–20.
4. Agostoni A, Aygoren-Pursun E, Binkley KE, et al. Hereditary and acquired angioedema: problems and progress: proceedings of the third C1 esterase inhibitor deficiency workshop and beyond. J Allergy Clin Immunol 2004;114:S51–131. http://dx.doi.org/10.1016/j.jaci.2004.06.047. pii:S0091674904017579.
5. Frank MM. 8. Hereditary angioedema. J Allergy Clin Immunol 2008;121: S398–401. http://dx.doi.org/10.1016/j.jaci.2007.07.057 [quiz: S419], pii: S0091-6749(07)01463-7.
6. Frank MM, Atkinson JP. Homozygous C1 inhibitor deficiency: the conclusion of a long search. J Allergy Clin Immunol 2006;118:1327–9. http://dx.doi.org/10.1016/j. jaci.2006.08.040. pii:S0091-6749(06)02010-0.
7. Cicardi M, Agostoni A. Hereditary angioedema. N Engl J Med 1996;334:1666–7. http://dx.doi.org/10.1056/NEJM199606203342510.

8. Cugno M, Nussberger J, Cicardi M, et al. Bradykinin and the pathophysiology of angioedema. Int Immunopharmacol 2003;3:311–7. http://dx.doi.org/10.1016/S1567-5769(02)00162-5. pii:S1567-5769(02)00162-5.

9. Ghebrehiwet B. The complement system. Mechanisms of activation, regulation and role in innate immunity. In: Greaves MV, Kaplan AP, editors. Urticaria and angioedema. New York: Marcel Dekker; 2004. p. 73–118.

10. Kaplan AP. Enzymatic pathways in the pathogenesis of hereditary angioedema: the role of C1 inhibitor therapy. J Allergy Clin Immunol 2010;126:918–25. http://dx.doi.org/10.1016/j.jaci.2010.08.012. pii:S0091-6749(10)01197-8.

11. Bork K, Frank J, Grundt B, et al. Treatment of acute edema attacks in hereditary angioedema with a bradykinin receptor-2 antagonist (Icatibant). J Allergy Clin Immunol 2007;119:1497–503. http://dx.doi.org/10.1016/j.jaci.2007.02.012. pii:S0091-6749(07)00379-X.

12. Tedesco F, Bulla R, Fischetti F. Terminal complement complex: regulation of formation and pathophysiological functions. In: Szebeni J, editor. The complement system. Boston: Kluwer Academic Publishers; 2004. p. 97–127.

13. Bossi F, Fischetti F, Pellis V, et al. Platelet-activating factor and kinin-dependent vascular leakage as a novel functional activity of the soluble terminal complement complex. J Immunol 2004;173:6921–7.

14. Avirutnan P, Punyadee N, Noisakran S, et al. Vascular leakage in severe dengue virus infections: a potential role for the nonstructural viral protein NS1 and complement. J Infect Dis 2006;193:1078–88. pii:10.1086/500949.

15. Nielsen EW, Johansen HT, Hogasen K, et al. Activation of the complement, coagulation, fibrinolytic and kallikrein-kinin systems during attacks of hereditary angioedema. Immunopharmacology 1996;33:359–60.

16. Ghebrehiwet B, Lim BL, Peerschke EI, et al. Isolation, cDNA cloning, and overexpression of a 33-kD cell surface glycoprotein that binds to the globular "heads" of C1q. J Exp Med 1994;179:1809–21.

17. Joseph K, Ghebrehiwet B, Peerschke EI, et al. Identification of the zinc-dependent endothelial cell binding protein for high molecular weight kininogen and factor XII: identity with the receptor that binds to the globular "heads" of C1q (gC1q-R). Proc Natl Acad Sci U S A 1996;93:8552–7.

18. Herwald H, Dedio J, Kellner R, et al. Isolation and characterization of the kininogen-binding protein p33 from endothelial cells. Identity with the gC1q receptor. J Biol Chem 1996;271:13040–7.

19. Hasan AA, Zisman T, Schmaier AH. Identification of cytokeratin 1 as a binding protein and presentation receptor for kininogens on endothelial cells. Proc Natl Acad Sci U S A 1998;95:3615–20.

20. Joseph K, Ghebrehiwet B, Kaplan AP. Cytokeratin 1 and gC1qR mediate high molecular weight kininogen binding to endothelial cells. Clin Immunol 1999;92:246–55.

21. Colman RW, Pixley RA, Najamunnisa S, et al. Binding of high molecular weight kininogen to human endothelial cells is mediated via a site within domains 2 and 3 of the urokinase receptor. J Clin Invest 1997;100:1481–7.

22. Joseph K, Tholanikunnel BG, Ghebrehiwet B, et al. Interaction of high molecular weight kininogen binding proteins on endothelial cells. Thromb Haemost 2004;91:61–70. http://dx.doi.org/10.1267/THRO04010061. pii:04010061.

23. Hasan AA, Cines DB, Herwald H, et al. Mapping the cell binding site on high molecular weight kininogen domain 5. J Biol Chem 1995;270:19256–61.

24. Pixley RJ, Espinola RG, Ghebrehiwet B, et al. Interaction of high molecular weight kininogen with endothelial cell binding proteins uPAR, gC1qR and cytokeratin

1 determined by plasmon resonance (BiaCore). Thromb Haemost 2011;105(6): 1053–9.

25. Ghebrehiwet B, Lu PD, Zhang W, et al. Identification of functional domains on gC1Q-R, a cell surface protein that binds to the globular "heads" of C1Q, using monoclonal antibodies and synthetic peptides. Hybridoma 1996; 15:333–42.

26. Shariat-Madar Z, Mahdi F, Schmaier AH. Assembly and activation of the plasma kallikrein/kinin system: a new interpretation. Int Immunopharmacol 2002;2: 1841–9.

27. Mahdi F, Madar ZS, Figueroa CD, et al. Factor XII interacts with the multiprotein assembly of urokinase plasminogen activator receptor, gC1qR, and cytokeratin 1 on endothelial cell membranes. Blood 2002;99:3585–96.

28. Shariat-Madar Z, Mahdi F, Schmaier AH. Identification and characterization of prolylcarboxypeptidase as an endothelial cell prekallikrein activator. J Biol Chem 2002;277:17962–9.

29. Kaplan AP. Mechanisms of bradykinin generation. In: Greaves MW, Kaplan AP, editors. Urticaria and angioedema. 2nd edition. New York: Marcel Decker; 2009. p. 73–90.

30. Regoli D, Barabe J. Pharmacology of bradykinin and related kinins. Pharmacol Rev 1980;32:1–46.

31. Margolius HS. Tissue kallikreins structure, regulation, and participation in mammalian physiology and disease. Clin Rev Allergy Immunol 1998;16:337–49. http://dx.doi.org/10.1007/BF02737655.

32. Erdos EG, Sloane EM. An enzyme in human blood plasma that inactivates bradykinin and kallidins. Biochem Pharmacol 1962;11:585–92.

33. Sheikh IA, Kaplan AP. Studies of the digestion of bradykinin, lysyl bradykinin, and kinin-degradation products by carboxypeptidases A, B, and N. Biochem Pharmacol 1986;35:1957–63.

34. Yang HY, Erdos EG. Second kininase in human blood plasma. Nature 1967;215: 1402–3.

35. Davis AE 3rd. C1 inhibitor gene and hereditary angioedema. In: Volanakis E, Frank M, editors. The human complement system in health and disease. New York: Marcel Dekker, Inc.; 1998. p. 455–80.

36. Petersen SV, Thiel S, Jensen L, et al. Control of the classical and the MBL pathway of complement activation. Mol Immunol 2000;37:803–11.

37. Jiang H, Wagner E, Zhang H, et al. Complement 1 inhibitor is a regulator of the alternative complement pathway. J Exp Med 2001;194:1609–16.

38. Nussberger J, Cugno M, Amstutz C, et al. Plasma bradykinin in angio-oedema. Lancet 1998;351:1693–7.

39. Donaldson VH, Rosen FS, Bing DH. Role of the second component of complement (C2) and plasmin in kinin release in hereditary angioneurotic edema (H.A.N.E.) plasma. Trans Assoc Am Physicians 1977;90:174–83.

40. D'Orleans-Juste P, de Nucci G, Vane JR. Kinins act on B1 or B2 receptors to release conjointly endothelium-derived relaxing factor and prostacyclin from bovine aortic endothelial cells. Br J Pharmacol 1989;96:920–6.

41. Bossi F, Fischetti F, Regoli D, et al. Novel pathogenic mechanism and therapeutic approaches to angioedema associated with C1 inhibitor deficiency. J Allergy Clin Immunol 2009;124:1303–10.e4. http://dx.doi.org/10.1016/j.jaci.2009.08.007. pii: S0091-6749(09)01182-8.

42. Bhoola KD, Figueroa CD, Worthy K. Bioregulation of kinins: kallikreins, kininogens, and kininases. Pharmacol Rev 1992;44:1–80.

43. Duchene J, Lecomte F, Ahmed S, et al. A novel inflammatory pathway involved in leukocyte recruitment: role for the kinin B1 receptor and the chemokine CXCL5. J Immunol 2007;179:4849–56. pii:179/7/4849.
44. Gao BB, Clermont A, Rook S, et al. Extracellular carbonic anhydrase mediates hemorrhagic retinal and cerebral vascular permeability through prekallikrein activation. Nat Med 2007;13:181–8. pii:10.1038/nm1534.
45. Su J, Cui M, Tang Y, et al. Blockade of bradykinin B2 receptor more effectively reduces postischemic blood-brain barrier disruption and cytokines release than B1 receptor inhibition. Biochem Biophys Res Commun 2009;388:205–11. http://dx.doi.org/10.1016/j.bbrc.2009.07.135. pii:S0006-291X(09)01506-X.
46. Merino VF, Todiras M, Campos LA, et al. Increased susceptibility to endotoxic shock in transgenic rats with endothelial overexpression of kinin B(1) receptors. J Mol Med 2008;86:791–8. http://dx.doi.org/10.1007/s00109-008-0345-z.
47. Cruwys SC, Garrett NE, Perkins MN, et al. The role of bradykinin B1 receptors in the maintenance of intra-articular plasma extravasation in chronic antigen-induced arthritis. Br J Pharmacol 1994;113:940–4.
48. Maeda H, Wu J, Okamoto T, et al. Kallikrein-kinin in infection and cancer. Immunopharmacology 1999;43:115–28.
49. Cicardi M, Banerji A, Bracho F, et al. Icatibant, a new bradykinin-receptor antagonist, in hereditary angioedema. N Engl J Med 2010;363:532–41. http://dx.doi.org/10.1056/NEJMoa0906393.

Rare Disease Partnership
The Role of the US HAEA in Angioedema Care

Bruce L. Zuraw, MD[a,b,*], Sandra C. Christiansen, MD[a,c]

KEYWORDS

- Hereditary angioedema • Rare disease • Patient advocacy • Registry
- Biorepository

KEY POINTS

- Like other patients with rare diseases, those with hereditary angioedema (HAE) are frequently misdiagnosed and often poorly managed because of a lack of sufficient knowledge and familiarity with HAE by the treating physician.
- Partnering with a rare disease patient advocacy group can improve the visibility of a rare disease to potential patients and pharmaceutical companies.
- The United States Hereditary Angioedema Association (US HAEA) has partnered with its Medical Advisory Board (MAB) to improve the diagnosis and treatment of HAE.
- The US HAEA has played an important role in HAE clinical research and has developed mechanisms that will significantly contribute to the success of future clinical and translational research efforts in the area of nonallergic angioedema.

INTRODUCTION

HAE due to deficiency of C1 inhibitor (C1INH) is caused by mutations of the SERPING1 gene that encodes C1INH.[1] Affected patients experience recurrent episodes of cutaneous and mucosal angioedema that typically begin in childhood and recur throughout life. The frequency and severity of attacks are highly variable; however, many patients experience significant morbidity from attacks, and there is a substantial risk of mortality from laryngeal attacks.[2] There have been tremendous advances in the scientific and clinical understanding of HAE in the past 60 years, and these have led to the development of several safe and effective drugs that can treat acute attacks or prevent future swelling attacks.[3] Despite the enormous progress that has been made, the correct diagnosis is often missed or delayed for decades and many patients have difficulty obtaining access to effective treatments. A substantial fraction of the difficulties in properly diagnosing and treating HAE stems from the fact that it is a rare disease.

[a] Department of Medicine, University of California San Diego, 9500 Gilman Drive, La Jolla, CA 92014, USA; [b] Department of Medicine, San Diego VA Healthcare, 3350 La Jolla Village Dr., San Diego, CA 92161, USA; [c] Southern California Kaiser Permanente, 7060 Clairemont Mesa Blvd, San Diego, CA 92111, USA
* Corresponding author. 9500 Gilman Drive, Mailcode 0732, La Jolla, CA 92014.
E-mail address: bzuraw@ucsd.edu

Immunol Allergy Clin N Am 33 (2013) 545–553
http://dx.doi.org/10.1016/j.iac.2013.07.011
0889-8561/13/$ – see front matter Published by Elsevier Inc.

immunology.theclinics.com

Rare diseases, by definition, occur infrequently. Based on the National Institutes of Health (NIH) definition, a rare disease has a prevalence of fewer than 200,000 affected individuals in the United States or approximately 1 in 1650. The precise prevalence of HAE is unknown but is generally believed to be around 1 in 50,000 without any known differences in gender, ethnic, or racial susceptibility. Because of the rarity of HAE cases, most physicians are unfamiliar with the disease, and even those who recognize the disease frequently do not see enough patients to develop adequate expertise to most effectively treat their patients.

It is within this context that partnerships between patient advocacy groups and expert physicians have emerged to address the issues that present such a challenge for rare diseases.[4] This article reports how a group of HAE clinical investigators partnered with the US HAEA to drive progress toward improving the diagnosis and treatment of HAE in the United States.

HISTORY OF THE US HAEA

In 1999, a group of patients with HAE began to meet under the auspices of the National Organization of Rare Disorders. A personal family Web site belonging to one of these individuals was devoted to discussing HAE and became the informal chat site for these patients to discuss their struggles with HAE. This chat site began to attract attention from a group of other patients with HAE. This small group of patients decided to incorporate themselves into a nonprofit 501c3 patient advocacy organization, the US HAEA. Among the earliest activities of the US HAEA was to build and maintain its own Web site, HAEA.org, dedicated to helping patients with HAE with "care, compassion, and kindness."

The mission statement of the US HAEA notes that it is "dedicated to serving all persons with angioedema. The Association provides HAE patients and their families with a support network and a wide range of services including physician referrals, and individualized patient support. Our goal is to increase awareness of Hereditary Angioedema by providing patients and physicians with authoritative and readily accessible information. We are committed to advancing and conducting clinical research designed to improve the lives of HAE patients and ultimately find a cure" (http://www.haea.org/about/mission/).

Once organized as a nonprofit patient advocacy group, the US HAEA put together a team of patient service representatives to respond to the concerns and needs of patients with HAE who needed assistance. Over time, this patient services team has grown to 6 full-time employees, each covering a different region of the country. The patient services team is one of the unique ways that the US HAEA has been able to provide help and advice to its members. Each of the patient services team members is a patient or caregiver of a patient, enabling them to have a comprehensive understanding of the concerns of US HAEA members.

The membership of the US HAEA now exceeds 4500 people and continues to grow every week. In addition to the Web site, the US HAEA maintains an active social network presence, including a Facebook page and a Listserv. The US HAEA was also a founding member and an active force in Hereditary Angioedema International (HAEi), which is an umbrella organization of the world's HAE patient advocacy groups.

HAE MEDICAL ADVISORY BOARD

The first broad multi-institutional HAE collaborative investigator group in the United States was formed in late 2002 in response to an initiative by the Division of Clinical Research of the National Center for Research Resources (NCRR) of the NIH to promote research into rare diseases through the formation of therapeutic development networks (TDNs). NCRR defined a TDN as a not-for-profit organization constituted to promote advances in treatment of a disease or group of diseases and consisting of a group of experts who would work with pharmaceutical and patient organizations toward treatment advances.

The impetus for the formation of the HAE TDN was the failure, in September 2002, of a multicenter phase III clinical trial of plasma-derived C1INH for the treatment of HAE attacks. Some of the investigators believed that the failure of this study was a direct consequence of problems in the study design. The study design problems had been raised in prestudy investigator meetings; however, the sponsor had declined to correct the study design. These investigators therefore banded together to form an HAE TDN in order to give investigators a stronger voice in future HAE clinical study design.

The original goals of the HAE TDN were to (1) establish a national registry of patients with HAE; (2) promulgate clear practice guidelines for the diagnosis and treatment of HAE, including the development of patient- and practicing physician–directed outreach and referral programs; and (3) coordinate clinical trials in HAE to promote accelerated and improved trial results. Among its first actions, the HAE TDN reached out to the US HAEA and secured its support. The HAE TDN proceeded to review and help shape each of the HAE clinical trials that were conducted over the subsequent decade.

In 2008, the US HAEA approached the HAE TDN chairman about forming an MAB. The original goal of the HAE TDN had been met with the successful completion of multiple HAE clinical trials. As a result, the primary goal of the HAE TDN shifted toward improving HAE care in the United States. An integrated partnership with the US HAEA seemed to be the best path toward accomplishing this goal. An agreement was reached in which the HAEA MAB would operate as an independent parallel group within the umbrella of the US HAEA.

The Chair of the HAEA MAB was to be chosen by the US HAEA Board of Directors and subject to approval by a vote of the members of the HAEA MAB. The HAEA MAB Chair would then, in consultation with the executive leadership of the US HAEA, appoint the members of the MAB based on their expertise and leadership in the area of angioedema, as well as their focus on patient-centric care. Most of the members of the HAE TDN became members of this MAB, which subsumed the HAE TDN.

Based on their common goals, the US HAEA and the HAEA MAB have subsequently engaged in a vigorous, ongoing, and forward-looking partnership. The HAEA MAB holds quarterly meetings during which their agenda is developed and voted on. The group also interfaces with the US HAEA on multiple levels as described later.

In the remainder of this article, the authors describe how this partnership between the patient-run US HAEA and the physician-run HAEA MAB has impacted and improved angioedema care in the United States. Specifically, this partnership has led to improvements in HAE diagnosis, patient and physician education, patient care, clinical trial performance, and research opportunities.

IMPROVING HAE DIAGNOSIS

The diagnosis of HAE is often overlooked and frequently delayed. In the classic review of HAE by Frank and colleagues[5] in 1976, the average delay between onset of HAE symptoms and establishment of the correct diagnosis was 22 years. A sustained effort during the last 30 years to decrease this delay through physician education via lectures and articles aimed at the Allergy and Immunology community succeeded in shortening the delay in diagnosis to around 10 years (Zuraw, personal communication, 2013). Even this delay, however, remains far too long. The mortality rate from HAE has recently been documented to be far higher in patients lacking the correct diagnosis compared with those in whom the correct diagnosis had been made.[2] Exposing patients with HAE, including children, who are otherwise healthy to the risk of morbidity and even mortality from untreated angioedema attacks is unacceptable.

The US HAEA and HAEA MAB have developed several additional strategies to shorten this delay before the proper diagnosis is made. One strategy has been to more strongly emphasize patient recognition of the possible diagnosis of HAE. The US HAEA Web site is the top hit when searching for "angioedema" or "swelling" on many search engines, including Google and Bing. The Web site gets an average of 5000 hits per month, with 32% of the hits from new visitors. Working with the HAEA MAB, the US HAEA has included straightforward and accurate descriptions and tables about the various types of angioedema on the US HAEA Web site that can help patients discern whether they may have HAE. By combining Internet searches with accurate and nonbiased information, the authors expect that many patients with recurrent angioedema will self-identify themselves.

A confirmed diagnosis of HAE, however, requires laboratory testing. Once a patient with recurrent angioedema suspects that he/she may have HAE, that patient must be evaluated by a physician who is familiar with the disease in order to establish the final accurate diagnosis. The US HAEA maintains a geographic database of more than 1500 physicians who treat patients with HAE. Patients seeking to confirm a possible diagnosis of HAE are given the names and numbers of physicians in their area who are known to be familiar with HAE and can provide an appropriate medical workup.

Another way that the HAEA MAB and US HAEA work to improve the diagnosis of HAE is through a regularly recurring series of patient meetings (described in more detail in the education section later). Many patients who have been diagnosed with HAE have affected relatives who remain undiagnosed. During regional and national patient meetings, patients are urged to provide information about HAE and the US HAEA to family members, often leading to a diagnosis of HAE. Again, the US HAEA Web site and the Patient Services Team help these patients find physicians in their area who can establish the diagnosis.

PATIENT AND PHYSICIAN EDUCATION

A significant barrier to proper diagnosis and treatment of HAE is the lack of specific knowledge about the disease among most physicians and patients. Improving HAE education for both patients and physicians is thus a key step toward improving HAE care. The HAEA MAB and the US HAEA have devoted considerable time and resources to this task by conducting patient meetings and developing educational materials.

The US HAEA holds regular regional and national patient conferences. Regional conferences typically attract 150 to 250 patients and consist of a 1-day program. The national conferences attract nearly 800 patients and consist of a $1^{1}/_{2}$-day program. A significant amount of the time during these conferences is devoted toward educating patients about the disease. Programs typically include presentations about HAE by expert physicians and an open question-and-answer session between the patients and a panel of physician experts. Talks about important issues concerning insurance benefits and patient assistance programs are given by experts in these areas. Representatives from the pharmaceutical industry are also invited to present updates and exhibits. Patients are thus given a full range of information about the current HAE landscape that can help them navigate the health care system and make rational choices regarding their own treatment.

The individual members of the HAEA MAB are involved with multiple professional organizations, particularly within the field of Allergy and Immunology, and often speak about HAE at local, regional, and national meetings. In addition, the US HAEA maintains booths at the American Academy of Allergy, Asthma, and Immunology meeting; the American College of Allergy, Asthma, and Immunology meeting; and meetings conducted by regional allergy associations. These booths provide physicians with a variety of informational and educational materials about HAE and the US HAEA.

The US HAEA and the HAEA MAB together also produce online educational materials and videos about HAE. These materials and videos cover the entire range of HAE diagnosis and treatment and are available on the US HAEA Web site. Separate modules are geared for either patients or physicians. Physician educational material includes a variety of documents written by the HAEA MAB as well as continuing medical education video educational programs. The patient resources similarly include a wide range of written, video, and audio educational materials. These educational materials are updated on a regular basis to stay current with the most up-to-date diagnostic and management recommendations.

IMPACT ON CLINICAL TRIALS

Most rare diseases do not have available even a single drug that has been developed and approved specifically for use in that disease. That at least 5 different drugs have undergone clinical trials in the past decade for the rare disease HAE,[6–10] with 4 of them already approved, is remarkable. Although not directly involved in conducting any of these clinical studies, the US HAEA played several key roles in promoting these clinical trials and facilitating their success.

The first role of the US HAEA was to increase the interest of the pharmaceutical industry in developing drugs for HAE. Considering the enormous costs of developing a new drug, pharmaceutical companies need to have confidence that there will be a market for their drugs if they are approved. By identifying many new patients with HAE and building a large membership, the US HAEA was able to make the case to pharmaceutical companies that it was worthwhile to invest in the development of new drugs.

Second, the US HAEA was instrumental in the successful completion of multiple randomized clinical trials of new drugs for patients with HAE. Enrolling sufficient numbers of subjects with a rare disease into clinical trials is a daunting task that must to be met to complete the trials. Clinical trials for rare diseases often do not use a randomized design because of this difficulty.[11] The US HAEA mission statement acknowledges the importance of clinical research, and the organization stresses this to its membership. Working with the pharmaceutical companies and individual investigators, the US HAEA helped publicize the clinical trials. In addition, during day-to-day interactions with the patient community, the US HAEA patient services team provided information about ongoing local clinical trials, stressed the importance of clinical trials, and encouraged members to enroll. Because of the credibility that the US HAEA had established in supporting and providing service to their membership, they were able to play a pivotal role in helping the HAE clinical trials meet their enrollment targets.

IMPACT ON PATIENT CARE

Patient care includes proper diagnosis, development of an appropriate treatment plan, patient education, and access to effective treatment. As described earlier, the US HAEA maintains a comprehensive geographic database of physicians who treat patients with HAE and has referred many patients to local physicians who are familiar with HAE. In 2012, the US HAEA provided physician referrals to 2475 patients who were either looking for a diagnosis or a doctor with experience in treating patients with HAE. This referral activity has had a significant impact on improving the accuracy of HAE diagnosis and allowing knowledgeable physicians to develop management plans for known patients. The US HAEA also plays an important role in patient care by educating patients about their disease and the types of treatments available.

The US HAEA has played a more direct role, however, in assuring optimal treatment of patients during angioedema attacks. The US HAEA patient service team provides 7 days/week 24 hours/day telephone emergency support for patients with HAE. In practice, these service team members frequently field calls from patients with HAE who are experiencing acute angioedema attacks and require immediate medical assistance. They provide information to the patients concerning the closest emergency rooms, as well as whether or not the hospital is known to stock one of the effective acute treatments. Team members then call the emergency room to alert them that a patient will be arriving. When necessary, the patient services team member will also arrange for a telephone consultation between the emergency room physician and one of the members of the HAEA MAB. During 2012, the US HAEA patient services team handled 113 emergency calls from patients suffering severe, often life-threatening, HAE attacks.

Another crucial area in which the US HAEA provides important help to the patients involves insurance issues and enrollment in company assistance programs. Patients and physicians are frequently unaware of the details on how to best use health insurance to get coverage for HAE treatment. The US HAEA patient services team helps patients deal with their insurance companies and maximize their benefits, so that they may gain access to life-saving medications. In addition, the patient services team also helps patients avail themselves of the patient assistance programs that have been developed by the pharmaceutical companies when their insurance plan does not fully cover the HAE medication cost.

Most ambitiously, the US HAEA has begun a unique collaboration with investigators at the University of California San Diego (UCSD) to develop an Angioedema Center. This Center is designed to be a national reference Center for the diagnosis and treatment of HAE and other forms of nonallergic angioedema. The US HAEA provided the seed support for this Center, and US HAEA personnel also assist patients with travel and insurance issues related to being seen at the Angioedema Center. The Center will offer comprehensive patient education tools that will empower patients to achieve life-long health. Angioedema Center physicians will work with referring physicians to implement individualized treatment plans for the patients seen at the Center. As the Center develops, it will offer educational opportunities for physicians and nurses wishing to learn more about angioedema. The Angioedema Center will also become a focus of HAE research, participating in clinical trials and initiating both clinical and laboratory-based translational research. Ultimately, the US HAEA hopes to establish additional angioedema centers at several locations around the country.

Finally, the US HAEA has worked closely with the HAEA MAB to establish guidelines for the diagnosis and treatment of HAE. The US HAEA hosted an international consensus meeting that developed the first widely recognized criteria for the diagnosis of HAE with normal C1INH.[12] Similarly, guidelines for the management of HAE have been developed by the HAEA MAB and published on the US HAEA Web site (http://www.haea.org/professionals/an-approach-to-the-diagnosis-and-treatment-of-hereditary-angioedema/). These guidelines have been recently updated and expanded by the HAEA MAB and submitted for publication.

IMPACT ON RESEARCH OPPORTUNITIES

Ongoing research is critical to the process of developing new and improved diagnostic and therapeutic modalities for angioedema care. The US HAEA has therefore committed itself to fostering research. The major areas in which it has pushed the research agenda are described here. These efforts have been undertaken both on its own and in collaboration with the HAEA MAB.

Because research support depends on recognition of the importance of the problem being studied, the US HAEA and HAEi worked hard to establish a global HAE day. The US HAEA brought HAE to the attention of the US Congress and was able to obtain a Congressional Resolution establishing an annual HAE Awareness Day in the United States. This important day is used to hold numerous HAE-related events around the world to raise awareness of HAE among patients and physicians and for fundraising to support HAE services and programs, including research.

The US HAEA has also lobbied the United States Congress for increased HAE research funding on the federal level. In support of this goal, the president of the US HAEA testified before a Congressional committee in charge of Department of Defense medical research appropriations. In response, the Department of Defense has included HAE as one of its target diseases in its Peer Reviewed Medical Research Program for the past 2 years. The US HAEA is also working to increase research funding for HAE at the NIH.

The US HAEA President, who also serves as the President of the HAEi, is leading an HAEi initiative that will commit $300,000 to fund research grants in HAE. This program is specifically designed to encourage young investigators to pursue a career in HAE. The request for applications (RFA) for this research grant opportunity will be sent to HAE investigators throughout the world in August 2013. Applications will be reviewed and scored by an independent panel of experts. HAEi anticipates that 2 to 4 grants will be awarded during the next couple of years. Depending on the response, HAEi will consider whether or not to extend the program into future years as well.

The most important US HAEA research initiative has been to develop with UCSD investigators a comprehensive disease-specific patient registry and biorepository. After obtaining informed consent, patients provide detailed clinical information, including general medical history, past HAE history, quarterly HAE history updates, and individual angioedema attack data. The questionnaires are primarily completed online, and stored in a Health Insurance Portability and Accountability Act of 1996 (HIPAA) compliant fault tolerate manner without clinical identifiers. Random codes are used to link the clinical data to biorepository samples, including plasma, serum, and DNA. Investigators will have access only to the deidentified data and samples to protect confidentiality. The robust clinical registry will provide unique opportunities to investigate the natural history of HAE, as well as the safety and efficacy of different treatment regimens. Combining the registry data with the linked biorepository samples should open new opportunities to study the mechanisms and pathophysiology of HAE.

SUMMARY

Rare diseases provide unique challenges to medicine, both for clinical care and for research. To meet these challenges, a strategy of forming active partnerships between clinical investigators, patient advocacy groups, and industry has been proposed.[13,14] The power of this strategy has been demonstrated for cystic fibrosis and alpha1-antitrypsin deficiency.[15,16] The US HAEA developed its own unique model to grow into a large patient-run organization that provides support for its members while working to improve the future of angioedema care. By partnering with physicians who share its goals and the pharmaceutical industry, the US HAEA has been able to make a significant impact in angioedema care in the United States, improving the diagnosis, management, treatment, and education of patients with HAE while developing the research infrastructure that will power future advances in the area. This type of partnership yields a highly efficient use of resources and has the power and potential to overcome the limitations inherent in dealing with rare diseases. Because it is estimated that there are up to 8000 different rare diseases[17] affecting more than 25 million Americans,[18] this model of partnership has broad implications for human health.

REFERENCES

1. Zuraw BL. Clinical practice. Hereditary angioedema. N Engl J Med 2008;359(10): 1027–36.
2. Bork K, Hardt J, Witzke G. Fatal laryngeal attacks and mortality in hereditary angioedema due to C1-INH deficiency. J Allergy Clin Immunol 2012;130(3): 692–7.
3. Cicardi M, Bork K, Caballero T, et al. Evidence-based recommendations for the therapeutic management of angioedema owing to hereditary C1 inhibitor deficiency: consensus report of an International Working Group. Allergy 2012; 67(2):147–57.
4. Dunkle M, Pines W, Saltonstall PL. Advocacy groups and their role in rare diseases research. Adv Exp Med Biol 2010;686:515–25.
5. Frank MM, Gelfand JA, Atkinson JP. Hereditary angioedema: the clinical syndrome and its management. Ann Intern Med 1976;84:586–93.
6. Zuraw BL, Busse PJ, White M, et al. Nanofiltered C1 inhibitor concentrate for treatment of hereditary angioedema. N Engl J Med 2010;363(6):513–22.
7. Zuraw B, Cicardi M, Levy RJ, et al. Recombinant human C1-inhibitor for the treatment of acute angioedema attacks in patients with hereditary angioedema. J Allergy Clin Immunol 2010;126(4):821–7.e14.
8. Cicardi M, Banerji A, Bracho F, et al. Icatibant, a new bradykinin-receptor antagonist, in hereditary angioedema. N Engl J Med 2010;363(6):532–41.
9. Cicardi M, Levy RJ, McNeil DL, et al. Ecallantide for the treatment of acute attacks in hereditary angioedema. N Engl J Med 2010;363(6):523–31.
10. Craig TJ, Levy RJ, Wasserman RL, et al. Efficacy of human C1 esterase inhibitor concentrate compared with placebo in acute hereditary angioedema attacks. J Allergy Clin Immunol 2009;124(4):801–8.
11. Remuzzi G, Garattini S. Rare diseases: what's next? Lancet 2008;371(9629): 1978–9.
12. Zuraw BL, Bork K, Binkley KE, et al. Hereditary angioedema with normal C1 inhibitor function: consensus of an international expert panel. Allergy Asthma Proc 2012;33(Suppl 1):S145–56.
13. Watson MS, Epstein C, Howell RR, et al. Developing a national collaborative study system for rare genetic diseases. Genet Med 2008;10(5):325–9.
14. Groft SC. Fostering research partnerships: a perspective from The Office of Rare Diseases (ORD). Retina 2005;25(Suppl 8):S86.
15. Ashlock MA, Olson ER. Therapeutics development for cystic fibrosis: a successful model for a multisystem genetic disease. Annu Rev Med 2011;62: 107–25.
16. Walsh JW, Snider GL, Stoller JK. A review of the alpha-1 foundation: its formation, impact, and critical success factors. Respir Care 2006;51(5):526–31.

17. Heemstra HE, van Weely S, Buller HA, et al. Translation of rare disease research into orphan drug development: disease matters. Drug Discov Today 2009; 14(23–24):1166–73.

18. Behera M, Kumar A, Soares HP, et al. Evidence-based medicine for rare diseases: implications for data interpretation and clinical trial design. Cancer Control 2007;14(2):160–6.

Index

Note: Page numbers of article titles are in **boldface** type.

Immunol Allergy Clin N Am 33 (2013) 555–559
http://dx.doi.org/10.1016/S0889-8561(13)00076-3
0889-8561/13/$ – see front matter © 2013 Elsevier Inc. All rights reserved.

immunology.theclinics.com

United States Postal Service

Statement of Ownership, Management, and Circulation
(All Periodicals Publications Except Requestor Publications)

1. Publication Title
Immunology and Allergy Clinics of North America

2. Publication Number
0 0 6 - 3 6 1

3. Filing Date
9/14/13

4. Issue Frequency
Feb, May, Aug, Nov

5. Number of Issues Published Annually
4

6. Annual Subscription Price
$306.00

7. Complete Mailing Address of Known Office of Publication (Not printer) (Street, city, county, state, and ZIP+4®)

Elsevier Inc.
360 Park Avenue South
New York, NY 10010-1710

Contact Person
Stephen Bushing

Telephone (Include area code)
215-239-3688

8. Complete Mailing Address of Headquarters or General Business Office of Publisher (Not printer)

Elsevier Inc., 360 Park Avenue South, New York, NY 10010-1710

9. Full Names and Complete Mailing Addresses of Publisher, Editor, and Managing Editor (Do not leave blank)

Publisher (Name and complete mailing address)

Linda Belfus, Inc., 1600 John F. Kennedy Blvd. Suite 1800, Philadelphia, PA 19103-2899

Editor (Name and complete mailing address)

Pamela Hetherington, Elsevier, Inc., 1600 John F. Kennedy Blvd. Suite 1800, Philadelphia, PA 19103-2899

Managing Editor (Name and complete mailing address)

Adrianne Brigido, Elsevier, Inc., 1600 John F. Kennedy Blvd. Suite 1800, Philadelphia, PA 19103-2899

10. Owner (Do not leave blank. If the publication is owned by a corporation, give the name and address of the corporation immediately followed by the names and addresses of all stockholders owning or holding 1 percent or more of the total amount of stock. If not owned by a corporation, give the names and addresses of the individual owners. If owned by a partnership or other unincorporated firm, give its name and address as well as those of each individual owner. If the publication is published by a nonprofit organization, give its name and address.)

Full Name	Complete Mailing Address
Wholly owned subsidiary of	1600 John F. Kennedy Blvd., Ste. 1800
Reed/Elsevier, US holdings	Philadelphia, PA 19103-2899

11. Known Bondholders, Mortgagees, and Other Security Holders Owning or Holding 1 Percent or More of Total Amount of Bonds, Mortgages, or Other Securities. If none, check box ☑ None

Full Name	Complete Mailing Address
N/A	

12. Tax Status (For completion by nonprofit organizations authorized to mail at nonprofit rates) (Check one)
The purpose, function, and nonprofit status of this organization and the exempt status for federal income tax purposes:
☐ Has Not Changed During Preceding 12 Months
☐ Has Changed During Preceding 12 Months (Publisher must submit explanation of change with this statement)

PS Form 3526, September 2007 (Page 1 of 3 (Instructions Page 3)) PSN 7530-01-000-9931 PRIVACY NOTICE: See our Privacy policy in www.usps.com

---

13. Publication Title
Immunology and Allergy Clinics of North America

14. Issue Date for Circulation Data Below
August 2013

15. Extent and Nature of Circulation

			Average No. Copies Each Issue During Preceding 12 Months	No. Copies of Single Issue Published Nearest to Filing Date
a. Total Number of Copies (Net press run)			434	371
b. Paid Circulation (By Mail and Outside the Mail)	(1)	Mailed Outside-County Paid Subscriptions Stated on PS Form 3541. (Include paid distribution above nominal rate, advertiser's proof copies, and exchange copies)	257	234
	(2)	Mailed In-County Paid Subscriptions Stated on PS Form 3541 (Include paid distribution above nominal rate, advertiser's proof copies, and exchange copies)		
	(3)	Paid Distribution Outside the Mails Including Sales Through Dealers and Carriers, Street Vendors, Counter Sales, and Other Paid Distribution Outside USPS®	55	52
	(4)	Paid Distribution by Other Classes Mailed Through the USPS (e.g. First-Class Mail®)		
c. Total Paid Distribution (Sum of 15b (1), (2), (3), and (4)) ▲			312	286
d. Free or Nominal Rate Distribution (By Mail and Outside the Mail)	(1)	Free or Nominal Rate Outside-County Copies Included on PS Form 3541	36	35
	(2)	Free or Nominal Rate In-County Copies Included on PS Form 3541		
	(3)	Free or Nominal Rate Copies Mailed at Other Classes Through the USPS (e.g. First-Class Mail)		
	(4)	Free or Nominal Rate Distribution Outside the Mail (Carriers or other means)		
e. Total Free or Nominal Rate Distribution (Sum of 15d (1), (2), (3) and (4)) ▲			36	35
f. Total Distribution (Sum of 15c and 15e) ▲			348	321
g. Copies not Distributed (See instructions to publishers #4 (page #3)) ▲			86	50
h. Total (Sum of 15f and g) ▲			434	371
i. Percent Paid (15c divided by 15f times 100)			89.66%	89.10%

16. Publication of Statement of Ownership
☐ If the publication is a general publication, publication of this statement is required. Will be printed in the **November 2013** issue of this publication. ☐ Publication not required

17. Signature and Title of Editor, Publisher, Business Manager, or Owner

[signature]

Stephen R. Bushing –Inventory/Distribution Coordinator

Date
September 14, 2013

I certify that all information furnished on this form is true and complete. I understand that anyone who furnishes false or misleading information on this form or who omits material or information requested on the form may be subject to criminal sanctions (including fines and imprisonment) and/or civil sanctions (including civil penalties).

PS Form 3526, September 2007 (Page 2 of 3)

Printed and bound by CPI Group (UK) Ltd, Croydon, CR0 4YY

08/06/2025

01896873-0008